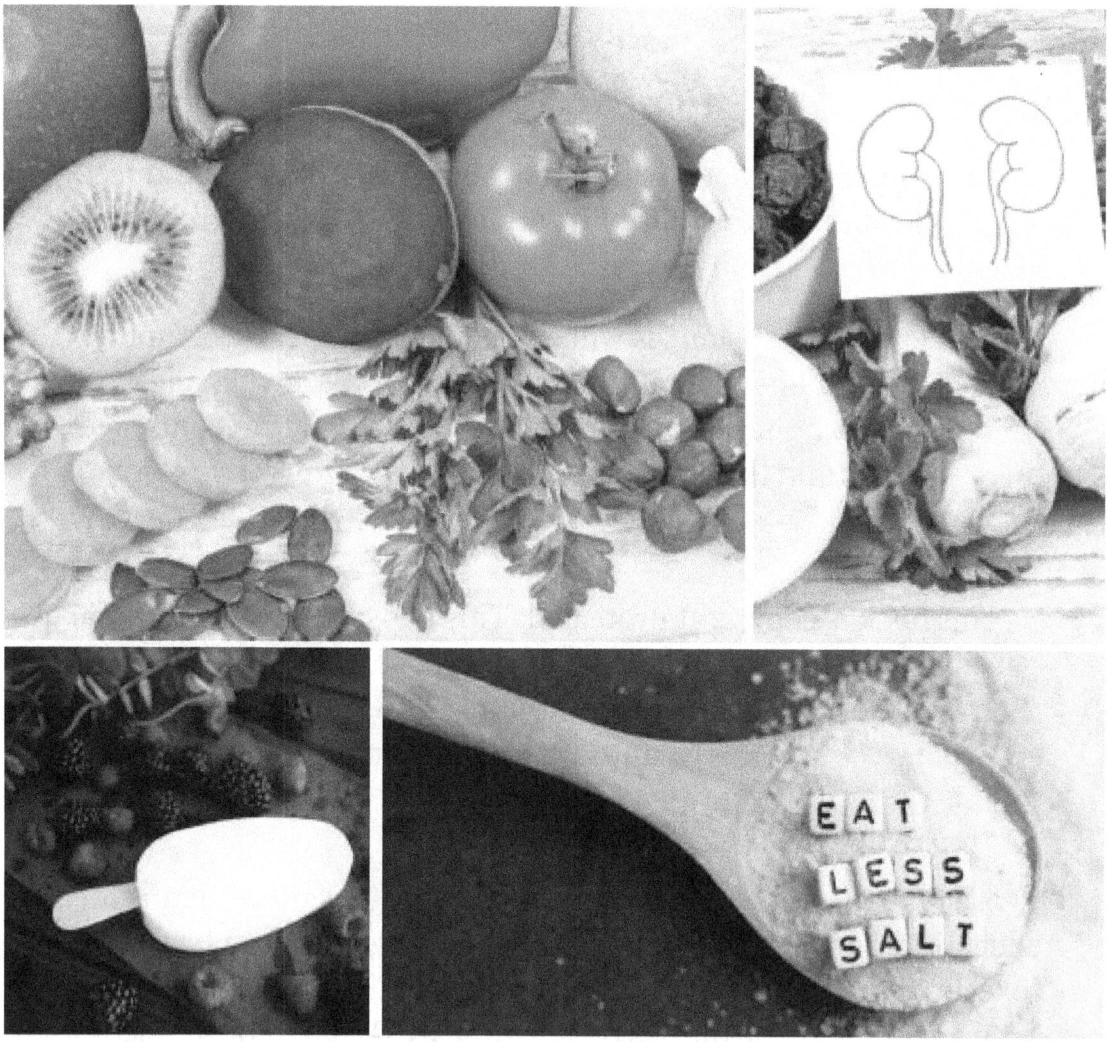

RENAL DIET

<u>COOKBOOK:</u>

150+ QUICK AND DELICIOUS RECIPES WITH LOW SODIUM, POTASSIUM, AND PHOSPHORUS FOR A HEALTHY LIFE. DISCOVER THE FIVE PROVEN TIPS TO SAFEGUARD AND MAINTAIN YOUR KIDNEYS' WELL-BEING

ANDREW MERRILL

TABLE OF CONTENTS

CHAPTER 6

LUNCH RECIPES

CHAPTER 7
DINNER RECIPES

CHAPTER 8
DESSERT RECIPES

INTRODUCTION

Your mission, should you choose to accept it, is to ensure that you minimize waste buildup in your kidneys. To do that, you need to watch what you eat, carefully preparing or arranging your meals so that you receive the required nutrition, minus all the unnecessary components.

This is where a renal diet becomes an essential component of your life.

Before delving deeper into the diet itself, let us look at some of the important substances that people with CKD need to manage.

Sodium

If you have been enjoying your pasta, nachos, pizzas, juicy steaks, lip-smackin' burgers, or practically any of your favorite savory food items, chances are that you have been consuming sodium. Why? Well, this mineral is commonly found in salt. Whether you use table salt or sea salt, you are going to find sodium in them.

If you have heard people claim that sodium is harmful to your body, then let me tell you that it is not entirely true. We need sodium in our bodies. The mineral helps our body maintain a balance in the levels of water within and around our cells. At the same time, it also maintains your blood pressure levels.

Surprised? You might have thought that sodium makes things worse, but there is a medical condition called hyponatremia, or "low blood sodium." When sodium levels drop to a low enough level, then you experience all the symptoms below:

- Weakness
- Nausea
- Vomiting
- Fatigue or low energy
- Headache
- Irritability
- Muscle cramps or spasms
- Confusion

In conclusion, sodium is essential for your body. But when you are on a renal diet, then you control the amount of salt that you add to your food. Since the kidneys are rather sensitive at this point, there is no need to exacerbate their condition by adding more sodium.

This might prove difficult for people since they are used to having salt as a flavoring ingredient in their foods. But that is why we are going to use recipes that are full of flavors that you will enjoy (more on that when we get started on the recipes).

Potassium

Potassium is one of those minerals that people might not think about too much as compared to calcium or sodium, but it nonetheless serves an important role in our body.

Apart from regulating fluids in the body, it also aids the body in passing messages between the body and the brain. Just like sodium, potassium is classified as an electrolyte, a term used to refer to a family of minerals that react in water. When potassium is dissolved in water, it produces positively charged ions. Using these ions, potassium can conduct electricity, which allows it to carry out some incredibly important functions. Take, for example,, the messages that are communicated between the brain and the body. These messages are sent back and forth in the form of impulses. But one has to wonder; what exactly creates those impulses? It's not like our body has an inbuilt electrical generator.

The answer lies in the ions. We have already established that sodium and potassium are both electrolytes and produce ions. The impulses are created when sodium ions move into the cells, and potassium ions move out of the cell. This movement changes the voltage of the cell, producing impulses. The way the impulses are created is similar to Morse code but takes place much faster (it has to for your body to react, manage processes, or perform tasks). When the level of potassium falls, the body's ability to generate nerve impulses gets affected.

Phosphorus

Finally, we have phosphorus. This mineral makes up about 1% of your body weight. That may not seem like a lot in actuality, but remember that our body consists of a lot of water. For this reason, oxygen makes up 62% of our total body weight, followed by carbon at 18%, hydrogen at 9%, and nitrogen at 3%. But guess which are the next two major elements in the human body?

- Calcium at 1.5%.
- Phosphorus at 1%.

So you see, even though phosphorus makes up just 1% of the total body weight, it is still a significant element.

What Is It Used for?

Let me put it this way. Phosphorus is one of the reasons you can smile wide. It is the reason your skin and other parts of the body are the way they are and do not just fall on the floor, like the way a piece of cloth might when you drop it. Phosphorus is responsible for the formation of your teeth and the bones that keep your body structure the way it currently is.

Pretty fantastic, isn't it? We often nominate calcium as the main element in the formation of teeth and bones, but forget the less popular, and often overlooked, partner element that helps with the same task.

However, the fact that phosphorus keeps our teeth and bones healthy is something people eventually discover. What they don't discover is that phosphorus also plays an important role in helping the body use fats and carbohydrates. The mineral is truly important for the everyday function of the body.

Fluids

Water sustains us. After all, 60% of the human adult's body is composed of water. This is why you might have heard of popular recommendations on how you should be having about eight glasses of water per day.

There is still a debate on exactly how much water is needed by an individual daily. But the fact remains; we need enough to avoid dehydration and keep the body functioning normally.

When you have kidney disease, you may not need as much fluid as you did before. The reason for this is that damaged kidneys do not dispose of extra fluids as well as they should. All the extra fluid in your body could be dangerous. It could cause swelling in various areas, high blood pressure, and heart problems. Fluid can also build up around your lungs, preventing you from breathing normally.

There is no measurement of how much fluid is considered as extra fluid. I strongly suggest that you should visit the doctor and get more information about fluid retention from him or her. The doctor will be able to guide you better and help you understand how much fluids you might require. The thing to understand here is that many of the foods that we eat, including fruits, vegetables, and most soups, have water content in them as well. Getting to know your kidney's ability to hold on to fluids will aid you in preparing or planning better meals for yourself.

The Renal Diet

When we follow the renal diet, we are going to make use of all the information about various components and minerals of foods to prepare a meal that is as ideal for your body as possible. One of the renal diet's main aims is to manage the intake of sodium, potassium, and phosphorus. At the same time, the renal diet focuses on consuming high-quality protein and limiting the consumption of fluids. I believe that knowing about what you should eat and what you shouldn't go a long way in finding out if there is anything in particular that you should avoid (due to allergies for example).

This book is designed to help. With over 150 recipes, plus tips and tricks, this book can help us tackle your new challenge together. It describes exactly what you can eat and what you should try to avoid.

CHAPTER 1:
<u>What is Renal Diet?</u>

How Does It Work?

A proper diet is necessary for controlling the amount of toxic waste in the bloodstream. When toxic waste piles up in the system along with increased fluid, chronic inflammation occurs, and we will be more prone to have cardiovascular, bone, metabolic, or other health issues.

Since your kidneys can't fully get rid of the waste on their own, which comes from food and drinks, probably the only natural way to help our system is through this diet.

A renal diet is especially useful during the first stages of kidney dysfunction and leads to the following benefits:

- Prevents excess fluid and wastebuildup
- Prevents the progression of renal dysfunction stages
- Decreases the likelihood of developing other chronic health problems, e.g. heart disorders
- Has a mild antioxidant function in the body, which keeps inflammation and inflammatory responses under control.

The above-mentioned benefits are noticeable once the patient follows the diet for at least a month and then continuing it for longer periods, to avoid the stage where dialysis is needed. The strictness of the diet depends on the current stage of renal/kidney disease. If, for example, you are in the 3rd or 4th stage, you should follow a stricter diet and be attentive to the food, which is allowed or prohibited.

So how exactly does the renal diet benefit you?

Preventing Diabetes and High Blood Pressure from Worsening

When you manage two of the biggest contributors of CKD, then you are delaying the effects of the disease greatly. You are getting out of a loop where either diabetes or high blood pressure makes the disease worse, further worsening either of the two conditions, which results in the disease entering a worse phase, and on it goes. This loop continues until it results in complete kidney failure.

Additionally, you might notice that your daily life becomes affected by CKD if you are not doing anything to manage the disease. You might find yourself losing focus on the things that you like, becoming less productive, and feeling too lethargic. You might also experience a greater degree of discomfort or exhaustion, even if you only have been walking at a normal pace.

A renal diet helps you avoid all the complications of diabetes and high blood pressure daily. Through careful planning, you might not feel as though your life has taken a heavy toll because of the disease. At the end of the day, you need to bring back as much normality in your life as possible, and a renal diet helps you with that.

Prevents Cardiovascular Problems

Because a renal diet manages various aspects of our health, including the consumption of sodium, potassium, and phosphorus, it aids in preventing cardiovascular risk factors from developing (Cupisti, Aparicio & Barsotti, 2007). When you manage the sodium content in your body, you also ensure that the levels of cholesterol are low. When you have too much cholesterol in your blood, then it tends to accumulate in the walls of your arteries. This process is called atherosclerosis and is a type of heart disease.

Why is the accumulation of cholesterol in the heart harmful?

Let's take an example to highlight this point. Imagine a highway with six lanes. On a busy day, the lanes are usually filled. You notice that vehicles can get by without facing any congestion, but it does not mean that they have empty roads to use. The roads are good to drive on because there are no accidents or anything to halt the smooth flow of traffic. Now imagine that the government decides that they have to perform maintenance on four of the six lanes. They block these lanes, and vehicles have to use two lanes for at least two miles. Imagine what would happen then. Think of the slow pace at which vehicles are going to move. In 2010, a reduction in road capacity caused a traffic jam in China that lasted for 12 days!

Now think of what happens when the same situation occurs in your body. Your arteries are the highways, and the blood that has to flow to various parts of the body are the vehicles. Cholesterol is the problem that blocks lanes and restricts the movement of blood. When enough blood does not reach your heart, then you begin to suffer from a myriad of problems, including chest pains and heart attacks.

Maintaining your cholesterol levels are important for healthy cardiovascular health. A renal diet ensures that you are avoiding foods that increase cholesterol.

Provides Essential Nutrients

The renal diet includes a lot of the good stuff and removes as much of the unnecessary stuff as possible. This means that the diet uses select ingredients to give you many vital nutrients in one meal. This ability of the diet to filter through various kinds of food to produce something extremely healthy for you is why it is popular among people with CKD who simply want to minimize the consumption of certain minerals.

Good Energy

One of the thoughts that zip through people's minds (I say 'zip' because it usually does not stay too long, and you are going to find out why) is if they might receive the right about of energy from a renal diet. We are all used to consuming a certain type of food that includes numerous minerals and essential components. The renal diet is going to cut many of those components out of your diet. It's like looking at a five-story building, deciding that the top three stories don't matter, and just decide to bulldoze the unwanted floors! Indeed, a renal diet is going to feel like an extreme diet, since you are going to suddenly cut down on a lot of foods. You are going to 'bulldoze' them from your daily meals.

However, with the kind of food that you are going to eat, you won't have to worry about energy. When you are on a renal diet, you can perform many physical activities that you might have thought you wouldn't be able to engage in after entering the diet.

You are going to get your energy from so many healthy and nutritious sources, as you will discover once you start reading through the recipes.

CHAPTER 2
Slowing Kidney Disease in 5 Steps

Having your kidneys function better for a longer period is one more day you don't have to worry about kidney failure. The more you slow down your CKD's progress, the fewer chances you have of finally looking for drastic kidney treatments. Some of the changes that you use for your kidneys also work to improve other organs in your body, such as your heart.

So, what are the tips that you need to follow to slow down kidney disease?

Tip #1: Maintain Your Blood Sugar in the Target Range

When you are checking blood sugar levels, you might find out that your blood sugar levels go through quite a few changes. It is not important to focus on these changes heavily when gauging the blood sugar levels, but they are important to know if you would like to get more details of your sugar levels. Before venturing further into understanding your glucose levels, I would like to first draw your attention to a particular measurement—mmol/L.

'Mmol' is short for millimole. A mole essentially calculates just how many atoms of a particular mineral or compound is present in a chemical process or reaction. A millimole is one-thousandth of a mole. The measurement is used to make precise calculations of the contents of fluids in our body, especially when it comes to blood sugar levels. The 'L' in mmol/L represent liters. What the measurement is trying to show you is the number of atoms of glucose or sugar (represented in mmol) is present in every liter of your blood. A typical adult will have anywhere between 4.7 to 5.5 liters of blood in their body. By using mmol/L, you get to know if you have high or low sugar content.

Tip #2: Exercise Regularly

If you were already consuming foods that are healthy, then it would also make sense if you were exercising regularly. Because regular physical activity will prevent weight gain and also regulate your blood pressure. But you should be careful about the amount of time you exercise or how much you exercise, especially if you aren't acclimatized to exercising. Don't overexert yourself if you are just getting started, because this would just increase the pressure on your kidneys and can also result in the breaking down of your muscles.

Tip #3: Be Careful When Making Use of Supplements

If you are consuming any supplements or any other herbal remedies, then you should be mindful of the amount you are consuming. Consuming an excessive amount of vitamin supplements, as well as any herbal extracts, can prove to be harmful to the functioning of your kidneys. You should talk to your doctor before you start taking any supplements.

Tip #4: Quit Smoking

Smoking causes damage to your blood vessels, and this, in turn, would reduce the flow of blood to and in your kidneys. When the kidneys don't receive sufficient blood, they won't function like they are supposed to. Smoking also tends to increase your blood pressure and can also cause kidney cancer, apart from damaging your lungs.

Tip #5: Over-the-Counter Medication

Whenever you are consuming any over-the-counter medications, then you shouldn't overdo it. Most of the common OTC medications tend to cause kidney damage if they are being consumed over a prolonged period of time. If your kidneys are healthy and if you consume these medicines for occasional minor ailments, then they don't pose a threat. But if you are taking them for any serious conditions like arthritis or chronic pain, then you should probably talk to your doctor before you start consuming them, and you should also keep monitoring the functioning of your kidneys. If you know that you are at risk of renal failure, then you should keep getting regular screening of the functioning of your kidneys for making sure that they are functioning normally. If you have diabetes or high blood pressure, t is advisable that you get your kidneys screened for any dysfunction.

CHAPTER 3
5 Stages of Kidney Disease

When you are diagnosed with chronic kidney disease, you will learn that kidney disease is an illness that takes a gradual approach to become worse. As it progresses from stage one to stage five, you'll find that it is very similar to completing different levels of a video game. Only, it's less fun, since the higher the level, the worse the disease. It is indeed something you should try your best to avoid.

Kidneys don't necessarily both fail at the same rate, either. Fortunately, if chronic kidney disease is caught early enough, it can be treated, and the process slowed down, allowing you to stay healthy for longer. Since there are five different stages of kidney disease, it is very important to identify how far your condition has progressed. If you know what stage of kidney disease you have, you can learn how to manage and treat it better, which will also aid in your overall well-being.

The NKF (National Kidney Foundation) has designed a guideline to help doctors identify the various stages of kidney disease in patients. Only when a doctor diagnoses a patient at a particular stage will he/ she be able to prescribe the best possible treatment options.

Even though doctors may run several tests on potential kidney disease patients, they usually make use of the glomerular filtration rate (GFR) to measure kidney function. Most importantly, the GFR is also used to depict what stage the patient is currently in. It is measured by using a math formula, an individual's race, gender, and age, as well as serum creatinine. The doctor will use blood tests to test GFR, particularly creatinine in the blood. If your kidneys are not working properly, there will be more creatinine in the blood, which will establish what stage of kidney disease you have.

Basic treatment options for stages one to five include regular check-ups with your specialist, along with scheduled tests to check the protein and serum creatinine in your urine and blood. When you are first diagnosed, your doctor will advise you to follow a healthy diet and give you prescription medication. As a kidney disease patient, you are advised to integrate different grains, fruits, vegetables, and food that is both low in saturated fat and moderate in fat content. You should also limit refined sugar, sodium, cholesterol, and of course, potassium, and phosphorus in your diet. If you are classified as either overweight or obese, you have to follow a diet plan that will also help you lose excess weight. Protein must only be consumed in moderation.

Monitoring blood pressure is also critical to managing chronic kidney disease. For patients with diabetes, it should be 125/75 for non-diabetics with non-proteinuria patients, 130/85, and for non-diabetics patients diagnosed with proteinuria, 125/75. Your blood sugar levels and diabetes must always be under control to ensure your kidneys won't become more damaged. Kidney patients are also advised to incorporate daily exercise as part of a healthy balanced lifestyle.

Stage One

Stage one kidney disease refers to a normal to high stage of chronic kidney disease with a glomerular filtration rate: GFR > 90 mL/min.

This is the earliest stage of chronic kidney disease that someone can be diagnosed with, which is usually the case when you have some kidney damage combined with a normal to high GFR that is higher than 90 ml per minute. When a doctor diagnoses you with stage one kidney disease, there are barely, if any, symptoms indicating that you have kidney issues.

The truth is, even though you have stage one kidney disease, your kidneys may still work efficiently. Even though the kidneys aren't functioning at their full capacity during this first stage, they can still function properly. Most people don't even realize they have any kidney problems when they are first diagnosed with stage one. This is often discovered when a person is testing for other potential health issues, such as diabetes, hypertension, or are getting a general blood test done. Given that diabetes and hypertension are the two leading contributing causes of kidney disease, testing for either will give your doctor an accurate result on whether or not you have stage one kidney disease.

So, although you can't always personally tell whether you have stage one kidney disease, your body may display some signs that could help you identify it. Symptoms that raise red flags include having blood or protein present in the urine or having higher urea or creatinine levels in your blood. All stages of kidney disease can be picked up by doctors with a CT scan, ultrasound, MRI, and contrast X-ray.

Stage Two

Stage two kidney disease is a mild type of chronic kidney disease, with a glomerular filtration rate: GFR = 60-89 mL/min.

Patients who have been diagnosed with stage two kidney disease have a mild case of kidney disease, which means they have a slightly higher decreased GFR. Still, just like with stage one, there may be no symptoms present. Stage two kidney disease is diagnosed the same way stage one is diagnosed.

Stage Three

Stage three kidney disease include types A and B. These are moderate types of chronic kidney disease, with a glomerular filtration rate:

- 3A = GFR = 45-59 mL/min

- 3B = GFR = 30-44 mL/min

Stage three kidney disease is considered to be a level of moderate damage inflicted on the kidneys. People with stage three kidney disease can be diagnosed as either type A or type B. Since stage three is halfway to stage five, meaning your kidneys' damage has increased, you are more prone to thebuildup of waste products in the blood, which causes uremia. During this stage, the patient is also more prone to developing complications due to their level of kidney disease, including anemia, hypertension, and bone disease.

Symptoms of stage three kidney disease include fluid retention, edema, kidney pain at the back of the kidneys, fatigue, urination changes, muscle cramps in the legs, as well as sleep issues.

If you've been diagnosed with stage three kidney disease or have progressed to this point, you should consult a nephrologist or kidney specialist, and not a general practitioner. A nephrologist will advise and help a patient manage treatment options for stage three, four, and five, if not earlier.

Although the renal diet is one of the best treatment options for all kidney disease patients, it is also recommended to consult a dietician. You can ask your nephrologist to advise you on finding the right dietician who you can consult about the renal diet for your specific case of kidney disease.

With stage one and two kidney disease, diet rules are quite simple, but with stage three to five, you will be advised to follow a stricter diet, as we'll discuss later.

This includes eating only high-quality potassium and proteins, should your blood levels be above normal. It also includes grains, fruits, vegetables, low-phosphorus, sodium, and calcium foods, decreased saturated fats, and consuming water-soluble vitamins, including vitamins C and B.

Your nephrologist will also provide you with the right medication prescriptions to manage your symptoms, as well as the progression of the disease.

Stage Four

Stage four kidney disease is a severe type of chronic kidney disease, with a glomerular filtration rate: GFR = 15-29 mL/min.

Stage four chronic kidney disease is the last level a patient reaches before he/she reaches level five, which is kidney failure. Stage four is an advanced level, with a severe decline in GFR. In most cases, stage four requires patients to be placed on the kidney transplant list, as well as permanent dialysis.

At this point, the functioning of the kidneys are at a minimum, and waste products are prone to accumulate in the blood. This causes worsened uremia, which can cause hypertension, anemia, bone disease, as well as heart disease.

Symptoms include fatigue, urination changes, kidney pain in the back, nausea, vomiting, fluid retention, muscle cramping, sleep issues, taste changes, bad breath, impaired concentration, loss of appetite, and even nerve problems.

A nephrologist must monitor kidney patients that have progressed to this stage, and take the necessary measures, including tests, medication, and dialysis to help patients manage this advanced level of kidney disease. At this point, patients are also likely to be hospitalized, depending on the severity of their condition.

Final treatment options for stage four include hemodialysis, peritoneal dialysis (PD), and a kidney transplant.

Stage Five

Stage five kidney disease is an end-stage type of chronic kidney disease, with a glomerular filtration rate: GFR < 15 mL/min.

This stage of kidney disease is also known as the end-stage of renal disease (ESRD), where you have reached a GFR of 15 mL/min or less. At this point, your condition has advanced to a point where your kidneys have lost nearly all of their ability to function. Reaching stage five, weekly dialysis, or finding a kidney donor to get a kidney transplant as soon as possible is non-negotiable.

At this stage, your kidneys aren't able to remove fluids or waste properly, which causes a dense buildup of toxins in the blood. This causes the body to have symptoms all over, causing one to feel very sick. Symptoms of stage five include headaches, fatigue, itching, loss of appetite, nausea, vomiting, muscle cramps, tingling in the nerves, skin discoloration, as well as increased skin pigmentation.

If you've reached stage five and haven't consulted a nephrologist, you have to do so immediately. All stage five patients must go for dialysis weekly, if not several times weekly, and be placed on the kidney transplant list to find a kidney donor. This must be done sooner than later, as the risk of fatality from stage five is quite high.

CHAPTER 4
<u>What You Can Eat and What You Should Avoid in Renal Diet</u>

Foods that you eat daily need to be regularly monitored. To encourage overall wellness, you need to take in less sodium, potassium, and phosphorus. Also, you need to eat more high-quality protein and lower your fluid uptake. Here is a detailed list of foods to eat and to avoid, which will make it easier for you to choose your next meal.

High in Sodium Foods That You Need to Avoid

- Different meats and sausages: chicken, pork, and cuts that have been preserved, smoked, or cured
- Fishes and seafood that are preserved
- Frozen dinners or packed dinners
- Canned food items like pasta or soup
- Salted nuts
- Salted and canned beans
- Buttermilk
- Cheese, cheese products, processed cottage cheese
- Quick bread and bread with extra salt
- Salted rolls
- Biscuits and pancakes made by self-rising flour or their mixes
- Salted crackers
- The dough of pasta, potatoes, and rice that is processed and packaged
- Vegetables and vegetable juices in cans
- Salted regular pickles as well as olives and other pickled vegetables
- Vegetables made with pork products
- The dough of hash browns and scalloped potatoes, which are processed and packaged
- Quick pasta meals
- Processed ketchup
- Processed and salted mustard
- Processed salsa
- Dehydrated or regular soups in cans
- Processed or regular broths
- Cup noodles processed and salted ramen mixes
- Soy sauce
- Seasoning salts
- Marinades that are salted
- Salad dressings in bottles, processed or regular
- Salad dressings with bacon
- Salted butter and margarine
- Instant custard or pudding
- Ready-to-eat cakes

Low in Sodium Foods That Should Be Taken Instead

- Fresh and frozen portions of lamb, poultry, beef, fish, shrimp, pork
- Fish and poultry, water and oil-packed, and drained; canned fish labeled as low sodium
- Eggs/egg substitutes
- Dried peas and not canned beans
- Low sodium peanut butter, almond, rice, or coconut milk, plant-based yogurts
- Low sodium cream cheese and low sodium cheeses like Parmesan and ricotta
- Ready-to-eat cereals
- Rolls and bread that are not salted
- Almond, coconut, whole-wheat, low sodium plain and all-purpose white flour; low sodium corn and tortillas
- Low sodium breadsticks, crackers, unsalted popcorn, and chips
- Pasta and rice cooked without salt and low sodium noodles
- Frozen or fresh vegetables, low sodium canned vegetables without seasoning or sauce
- Low sodium vegetable juices, V-8, and low sodium tomato juice
- Low sodium pickles
- Fresh potatoes or unsalted and unseasoned frozen French fries and mashed potatoes
- Fresh and frozen canned fruits, dried fruits
- Low sodium salsa
- Low sodium soups that are canned
- Homemade broths made without any salt, and fresh ingredients
- Homemade pasta without any salt
- Low sodium soy sauce
- Low sodium seasoning and marinades
- Low sodium salad dressings
- Low sodium mayonnaise
- Unsalted butter and margarine, vegetable oils
- Homemade ketchup that is unsalted
- Unsalted mustard

High in Potassium Foods That You Need to Avoid

- Cooked spinach, artichokes, okra, broccoli, beets, fried onions, and sweet potato
- Bananas, avocados, honeydew, mango, orange, pomegranate, prune, pumpkin, coconut, and cantaloupe
- Buttermilk and shakes
- Beans, either baked or refried
- Legumes, like lentils
- Nuts, like walnuts and raisins
- Granola
- Whole grains and bran
- Fast foods, like french fries and other salty foods
- Processed meats
- Vegetable juices
- Processed sauces, like tomato sauce
- Fruit juices such as pomegranate juice, prune juice
- Creamed soups
- Yogurt, frozen and regular
- Ice creams
- Chocolate sweet dishes

Low in Potassium Foods That You Need to Eat Instead

- Asparagus, kale, broccoli, cucumber, zucchini, carrots, cabbage, bell pepper, eggplant, garlic, and lettuce
- Apples, grapes, pineapple, peaches, plum, all berries, watermelon
- Rice milk
- Greens beans and snow peas
- White rice and bread that is not whole
- Dried cranberries
- Unsalted popcorn
- Hash browns and mashed potatoes made up of leached potatoes
- Low sodium tomato and V-8 juice
- Unsalted sauces and apple sauce
- Unsalted noodles and pasta
- Non-dairy creams
- Sherbet
- Lemon and vanilla flavors instead of chocolate

High in Phosphorus Foods That Need to Be Avoided

- Some Vegetables
- Some Fruits
- Parts of chicken and other poultry
- Ham and other pork products
- Hunted animals
- Some Seafood
- Plain Bread
- Tortillas
- Muffins
- Some pasta
- Some types of rice
- Certain cheeses
- Milk
- Yogurt
- Ice cream
- Eggs
- Snacks

Low in Phosphorus Foods That Should Be Eaten Instead

- Celery, radishes, and baby carrots
- Apples, cherries, peaches, pineapples, blueberries, and strawberries
- Pot roast beef, sirloin steak
- Skinless chicken and turkey, breast and thighs
- Porkchop, mostly lean pork patty and pork roast
- Veal chop
- Wild salmon, mahi-mahi, king crab, lobster, snow crab, oyster shrimp, water, or oil-packed canned tuna
- Plain bread without salt, Italian bread, blueberry bread, sourdough bread, white bread, flatbread, wheat bread, pita bread, and cinnamon bread
- Flour tortillas, corn tortillas
- English muffins
- Macron, egg and rice noodles, spaghetti
- Couscous, long-grain white rice
- Cottage, blue, feta, Parmesan, and cream cheese
- Almond, soy, and rice milk
- Non-dairy creamer
- Sorbet
- Pasteurized egg whites
- Unsalted popcorn

Kidney-Friendly Protein Options Which Are Included in the Overall Diet

- Lean beef and turkey
- Meat substitutes, like tofu and veggie sausage
- Skinless chicken breast and thigh
- Salman, trout, mackerel fish, and shrimp
- Pork chops
- Cottage cheese
- Pasteurized eggs
- Greek yogurt
- Shakes made with rice, almond, coconut, or soy milk

Kidney-Friendly Fluid Options Which Are Included in This Diet

- Fruits like apples, cherries, grapes, berries, peaches, plums
- Vegetables such as zucchini, cucumber, broccoli, cauliflower, cabbage, bell peppers, carrots, celery, lettuce, and eggplant
- Tea and coffee
- Gelatin
- Ice cubes
- Fruit juices
- Popsicles
- Milk substitutes
- Sherbet
- Low sodium soups

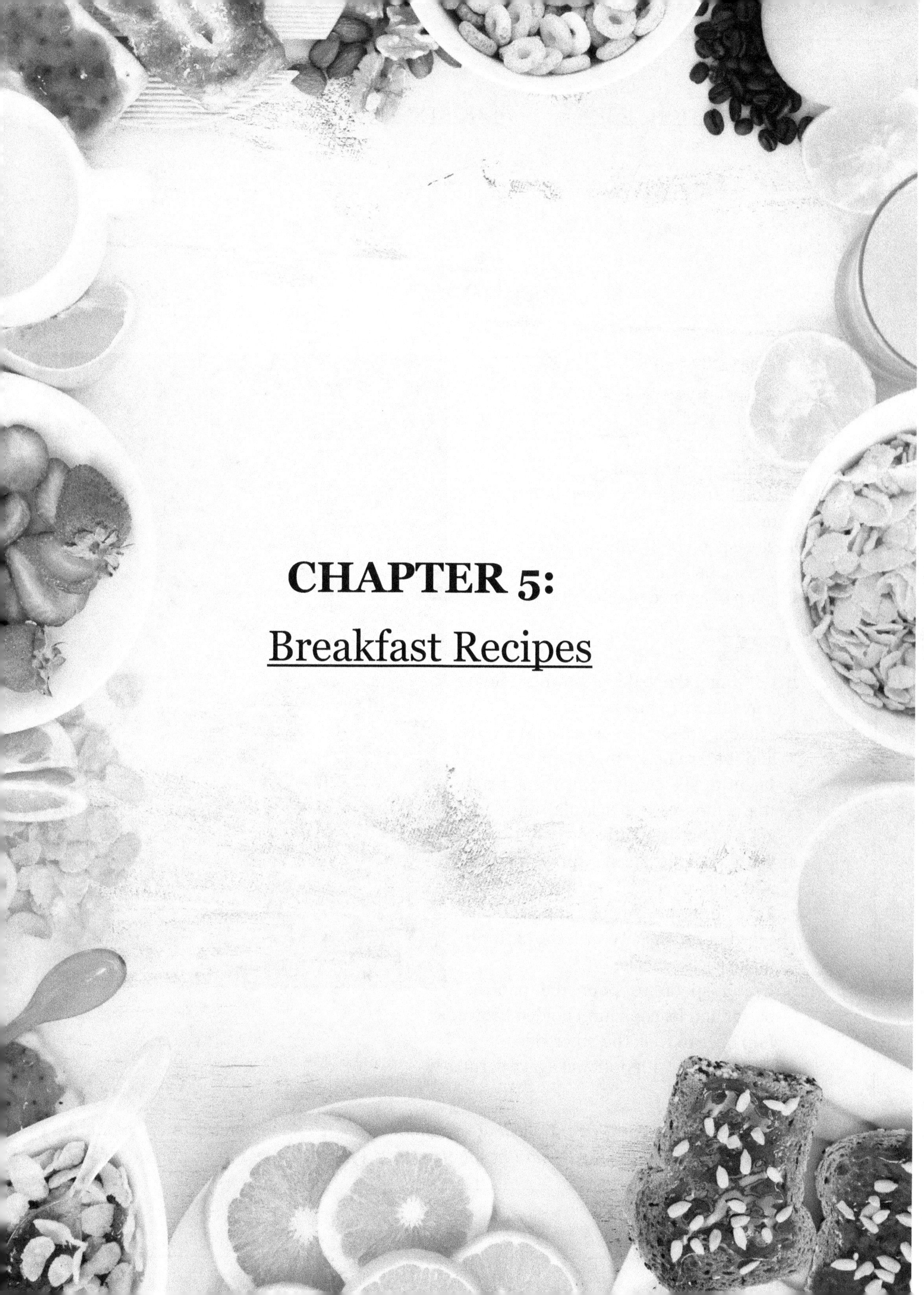

CHAPTER 5:

Breakfast Recipes

AMERICAN BLUEBERRY PANCAKES

INGREDIENTS:

- 1 ½ cups of all-purpose flour, sifted
- 1 cup of buttermilk
- 3 tablespoons of sugar
- 2 tablespoons of unsalted butter, melted
- 2 teaspoon of baking powder
- 2 eggs, beaten
- 1 cup of canned blueberries, rinsed

DIRECTIONS:

1. Combine the baking powder, flour, and sugar in a bowl.
2. Make a hole in the center and slowly add the rest of the ingredients.
3. Begin to stir gently from the sides to the center with a spatula, until you get a smooth and creamy batter.
4. With cooking spray, spray the pan and place over medium heat.
5. Take one measuring cup and fill 1/3rd of its capacity with the batter to make each pancake.
6. Use a spoon to pour the pancake batter and let cook until golden brown. Flip once to cook the other side.
7. Serve warm with optional agave syrup.

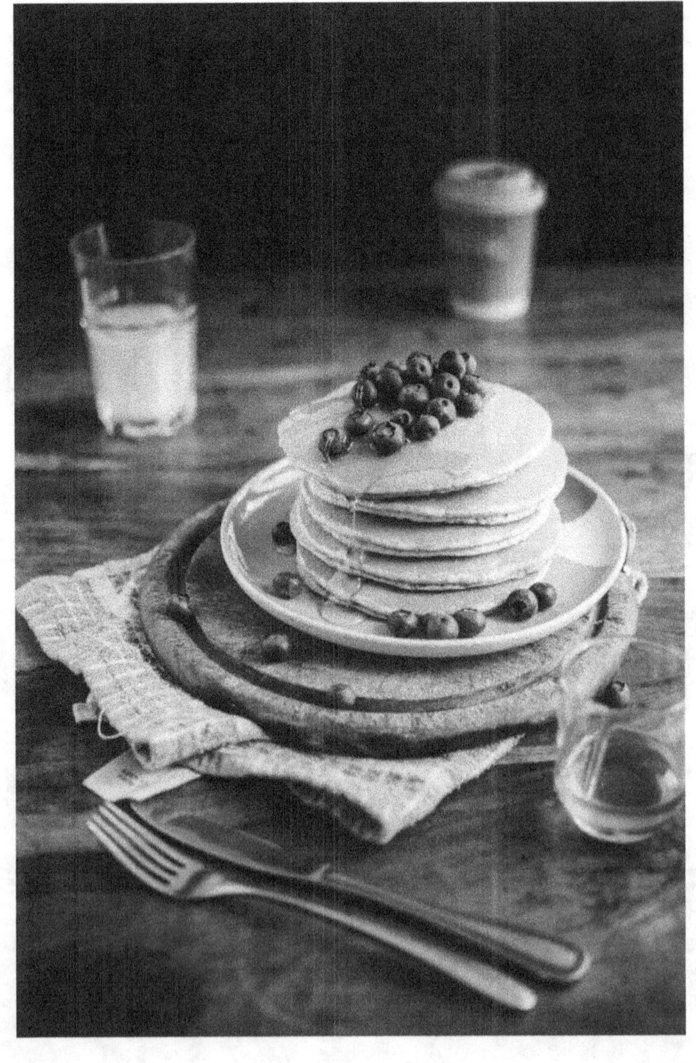

Nutrition: *Calories: 251.69kcal Carbohydrate: 41.68g Protein: 7.2g Sodium: 186.68mg Potassium: 142.87mg Phosphorus: 255.39mg Dietary Fiber: 1.9g Fat: 6.47g*

RASPBERRY PEACH
BREAKFAST SMOOTHIE

INGREDIENTS:

- 1/3 cup of raspberries (it can be frozen)
- 1/2 peach, skin and pit removed
- 1 tablespoon of honey
- 1 cup of coconut water

DIRECTIONS:

1. Mix all ingredients together and blend until smooth.
2. Pour and serve chilled in a tall glass or mason jar.

Nutrition: *Calories: 86.3kcal Carbohydrate: 20.6g Protein: 1.4g Sodium: 3mg Potassium: 109mg Phosphorus: 36.08mg Dietary Fiber: 2.6g Fat: 0.31g*

CAULIFLOWER WITH

MUSTARD SAUCE

INGREDIENTS:

- 1 head cauliflower, separated into florets
- 1/2 cup mayonnaise
- 1/4 cup Dijon mustard
- 1 cup sharp Cheddar cheese, shredded

DIRECTIONS:

1. Whisk the mayonnaise with the mustard and cheese in a bowl.
2. Add the cauliflower florets in boiling water in a pot and cook until they are tender.
3. Drain the cauliflower, then toss its florets with the mayo mixture.
4. Spread the cauliflower mixture in a baking pan.
5. Broil it for 5 minutes until the cheese is melted.
6. Serve fresh.

Nutrition: *Calories: 255 Total Fat: 19.9g Saturated Fat: 7.5g Cholesterol: 37mg Sodium: 582mg Carbohydrate: 11.7g Dietary Fiber: 2.2g Sugars: 3.8g Protein: 9.3g Calcium: 231mg Phosphorous: 97mg Potassium: 253mg*

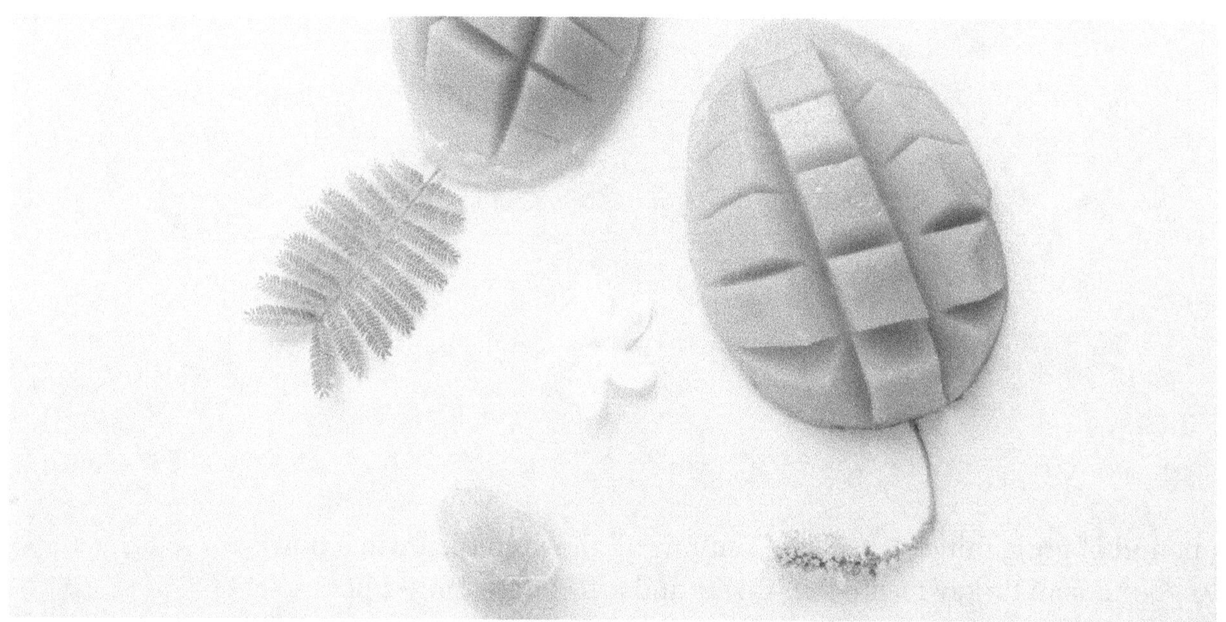

MANGO LASSI SMOOTHIE

INGREDIENTS:

- ½ cup of plain yogurt
- ½ cup of plain water
- ½ cup of sliced mango
- 1 tablespoon of sugar
- ¼ teaspoon of cardamom
- ¼ teaspoon cinnamon
- ¼ cup lime juice

DIRECTIONS:

1. Pulse all the above ingredients in a blender until smooth (around 1 minute).
2. Pour into tall glasses or mason jars and serve chilled immediately.

Nutrition: *Calories: 89.02kcal Carbohydrate: 14.31g Protein: 2.54g Sodium: 30mg Potassium: 185.67mg Phosphorus: 67.88mg Dietary Fiber: 0.77g Fat: 2.05g*

BREAKFAST MAPLE SAUSAGE

INGREDIENTS:

- 1 pound of pork, minced
- ½ pound lean turkey meat, ground
- ¼ teaspoon of nutmeg
- ½ teaspoon black pepper
- ¼ allspice
- 2 tablespoon of maple syrup
- 1 tablespoon of water

DIRECTIONS:

1. Combine all the ingredients in a bowl.
2. Cover and refrigerate for 3-4 hours.
3. Take the mixture and form into small flat patties with your hand (around 10-12 patties).
4. Lightly grease a medium skillet with oil and shallow fry the patties over medium to high heat, until brown (around 4-5 minutes on each side).
5. Serve hot.

Nutrition: *Calories: 53.85kcal Carbohydrate: 2.42g Protein: 8.5g Sodium: 30.96mg Potassium: 84.68mg Phosphorus: 83.49mg Dietary Fiber: 0.03g Fat: 0.9g*

PREPARATION: 5 MIN   **COOKING:** 5 MIN   **SERVINGS:** 2

SUMMER VEGGIE OMELET

INGREDIENTS:

- 4 large egg whites
- ¼ cup of sweet corn, frozen
- ⅓ cup of zucchini, grated
- 2 green onions, sliced
- 1 tablespoon of cream cheese
- Kosher pepper

DIRECTIONS:

1. Grease a medium pan with some cooking spray and add the onions, corn, and grated zucchini.
2. Sauté for a couple of minutes until softened.
3. Beat the eggs together with the water, cream cheese, and pepper in a bowl.
4. Add the eggs into the veggie mixture in the pan, and let cook while moving the edges from inside to outside with a spatula to allow raw egg to cook through the edges.
5. Turn the omelette with the aid of a dish (placed over the pan and flipped upside down and then back to the pan).
6. Let sit for another 1-2 minutes.
7. Fold in half and serve.

Nutrition: *Calories: 90kcal Carbohydrate: 15.97g Protein: 8.07g Sodium: 227mg Potassium: 244.24mgPhosphorus: 45.32mg Dietary Fiber: 0.88g Fat: 2.44g*

RASPBERRY OVERNIGHT PORRIDGE

INGREDIENTS:

- ⅓ cup of rolled oats
- ½ cup almond milk
- 1 tablespoon of honey
- 5-6 raspberries, fresh or canned and unsweetened
- ⅓ cup of rolled oats
- ½ cup almond milk
- 1 tablespoon of honey
- 5-6 raspberries, fresh or canned and unsweetened

DIRECTIONS:

1. Combine the oats, almond milk, and honey in a mason jar and place it into the fridge overnight.
2. Serve the next morning with the raspberries on top.

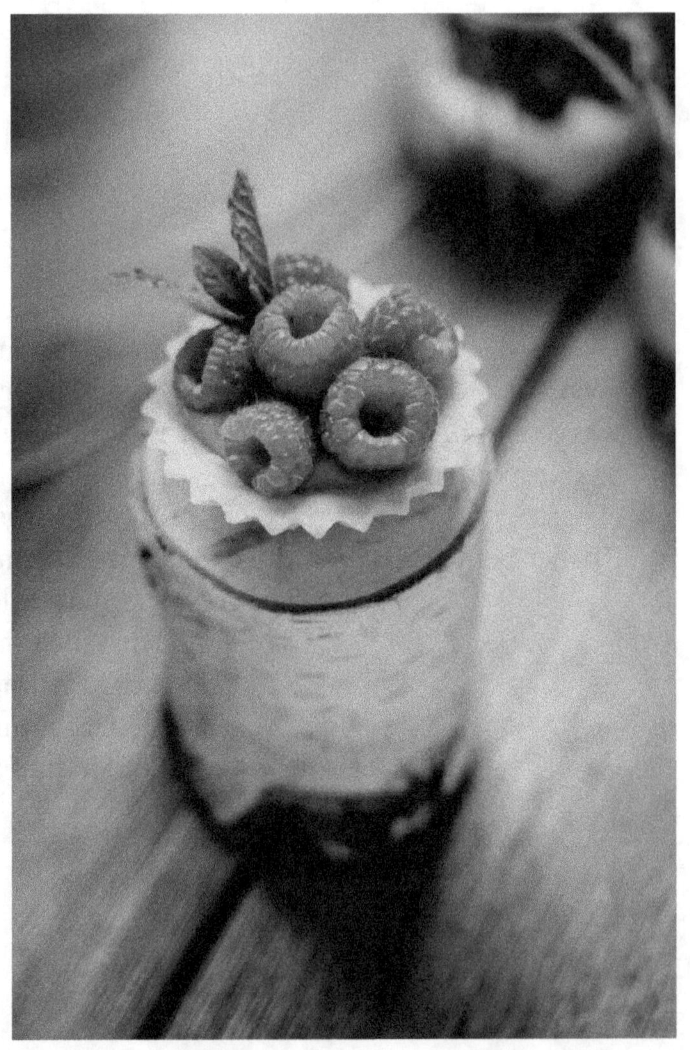

Nutrition: *Calories: 143.6kcal Carbohydrate: 34.62g Protein: 3.44g Sodium: 77.88mg Potassium: 153.25mg Phosphorus: 99.3mg Dietary Fiber: 7.56g Fat: 3.91g*

CRUNCHY CHICKEN SALAD WRAPS

INGREDIENTS:

- 8 ounces cooked shredded chicken
- 1 scallion, white and green parts, chopped
- ½ cup halved seedless red grapes
- 1 celery stalk, chopped
- ¼ cup Low-Sodium Mayonnaise (here) or store-bought mayonnaise
- Pinch freshly ground black pepper
- 4 large lettuce leaves, butter or red leaf

DIRECTIONS:

1. In a medium bowl, stir together the chicken, scallion, grapes, celery, and mayonnaise until well mixed.
2. Season the mixture with pepper.
3. Spoon the chicken salad onto the lettuce leaves and serve.
4. Ingredient tip One of the freshest kinds of butter lettuce you can buy is a hydroponic variety sold with the roots still attached. Most supermarkets carry these heads, and they are so fresh you might swear you could see dew on the leaves.

Nutrition: *Calories: 110 Total Fat: 3g Saturated Fat: 1g Cholesterol: 36mg Sodium: 61mg Total Carbs: 6g Fiber: 0g Sugar: 0g Protein: 13g*

TURKEY AND SPINACH SCRAMBLE ON MELBA TOAST

INGREDIENTS:

- Extra virgin olive oil – 1 teaspoon
- Raw spinach – 1 cup
- Garlic – ½ clove, minced
- Nutmeg – 1 teaspoon grated
- Cooked and diced turkey breast – 1 cup
- Melba toast – 4 slices
- Balsamic vinegar – 1 teaspoon

DIRECTIONS:

1. Heat a pot over a source of heat and add oil.
2. Add turkey and heat through for 6 to 8 minutes.
3. Add spinach, garlic, and nutmeg and stir-fry for 6 minutes more.
4. Plate up the Melba toast and top with spinach and turkey scramble.
5. Drizzle with balsamic vinegar and serve.

Nutrition: *Calories: 301 Fat: 19g Carb: 12g Phosphorus: 215mg Potassium: 269mg Sodium: 360mg Protein: 19g*

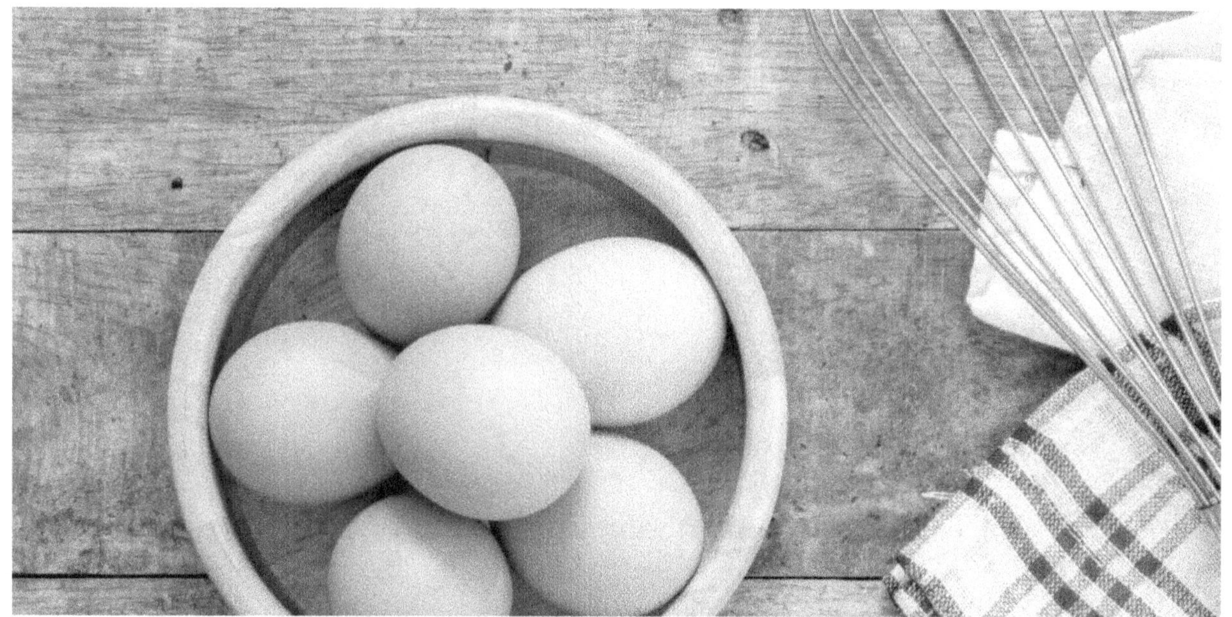

VEGETABLE OMELET

INGREDIENTS:

- Egg whites – 4
- Egg – 1
- Chopped fresh parsley – 2 tablespoons.
- Water – 2 tablespoons.
- Olive oil spray
- Chopped and boiled red bell pepper – ½ cup
- Chopped scallion – ¼ cup, both green and white parts
- Ground black pepper

DIRECTIONS:

1. Whisk together the egg, egg whites, parsley, and water until well blended. Set aside.
2. Spray a skillet with olive oil spray and place over medium heat.
3. Sauté the peppers and scallion for 3 minutes or until softened.
4. Over the vegetables, you can now pour the egg and cook, swirling the skillet, for 2 minutes or until the edges start to set. Cook until set.
5. Season with black pepper and serve.

Nutrition: *Calories: 77 Fat: 3g Carb: 2g Phosphorus: 67mg Potassium: 194mg Sodium: 29mg Protein: 12g*

MEXICAN STYLE BURRITOS

INGREDIENTS:

- Olive oil – 1 tablespoon
- Corn tortillas – 2
- Red onion – ¼ cup, chopped
- Red bell peppers – ¼ cup, chopped
- Red chili – ½, deseeded and chopped
- Eggs – 2
- Juice of 1 lime
- Cilantro – 1 tablespoon chopped

DIRECTIONS:

1. Turn the broiler to medium heat and place the tortillas underneath for 1 to 2 minutes on each side or until lightly toasted.
2. Remove and keep the broiler on.
3. Sauté onion, chili, and bell peppers for 5 to 6 minutes or until soft.
4. Place the eggs on top of the onions and peppers and place skillet under the broiler for 5-6 minutes or until the eggs are cooked.
5. Serve half the eggs and vegetables on top of each tortilla and sprinkle with cilantro and lime juice to serve.

Nutrition:*Calories: 202 Fat: 13g Carb: 19g Phosphorus: 184mg Potassium: 233mg Sodium: 7mg Protein: 9g*

CAULIFLOWER AND ASPARAGUS TORTILLA

INGREDIENTS:

- Asparagus – 2 cups
- Cauliflower – 2 cups
- Olive oil – 2 teaspoons
- Onion – 1½ cups
- Garlic – 1 clove
- Liquid egg substitute (low-cholesterol) – 1 cup
- Fresh parsley (finely chopped) – 2 tablespoons
- Salt – ¼ teaspoon
- Pepper (freshly ground) – ½ teaspoon
- Dried thyme leaves (crushed) – ¼ teaspoon
- Ground nutmeg – ¼ teaspoon

DIRECTIONS:

1. Start by chopping the asparagus and cauliflower into 1-inch pieces. Take the onion and chop it finely. Also, mince the garlic clove.
2. Take a microwave-safe bowl and place the chopped cauliflower and asparagus pieces into it. Add in 1 tablespoon of water and cover the dish.
3. After that, drain any excess water and set aside.
4. Microwave them for about 4-5 minutes. Make sure the veggies are slightly tender.
5. Place a saucepan over a high flame and pour the oil into it. Once heated, toss in the finely chopped onions.
6. Sauté the onions for about 6-7 minutes. Add in the minced garlic and sauté for 1 more minute.
7. Toss in the cauliflower, asparagus, egg substitute, salt, thyme, parsley, and nutmeg. Arrange them well over the egg substitute base.
8. Cover the saucepan, and cook for about 15 minutes on low heat.
9. Use a butter knife to loosen the edges of the prepared tortilla.
10. Take a microwave-safe serving platter and heat it for about 30-40 seconds.
11. Invert the tortilla onto the heated serving platter. Serve hot!

Nutrition: *Protein: 9g Fat: 3g Carbohydrates: 9g Sodium: 248mg Cholesterol: 0mg Potassium: 472mg Calcium: 68mg Phosphorus: 97mg Fiber: 3.88g*

BREAKFAST SMOOTHIE

INGREDIENTS:

- Frozen blueberries – 1 cup
- Pineapple chunks – ½ cup
- English cucumber – ½ cup
- Apple – ½
- Water – ½ cup

DIRECTIONS:

1. Put the pineapple, blueberries, cucumber, apple, and water in a blender and blend until thick and smooth.
2. Pour into 2 glasses and serve.

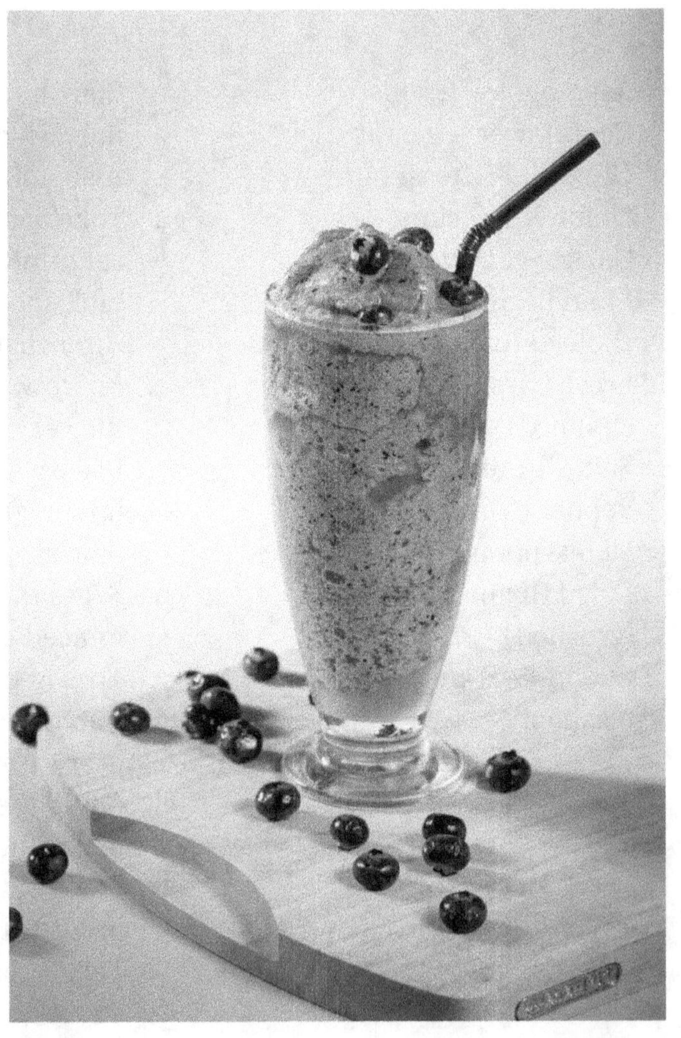

Nutrition: *Calories: 87 Fat: 3g Carb: 22g Phosphorus: 28mg Potassium: 192mg Sodium: 3mg Protein: 0.7g*

BUCKWHEAT AND GRAPEFRUIT PORRIDGE

INGREDIENTS:

- Buckwheat – ½ cup
- Grapefruit – ¼, chopped
- Honey – 1 tablespoon
- Almond milk – 1 ½ cups
- Water – 2 cups

DIRECTIONS:

1. Boil water on the stove. Add the buckwheat and place the lid on the pan.
2. Simmer for 7 to 10 minutes, in low heat. Check to ensure water does not dry out.
3. Remove and set aside for 5 minutes, do this when most of the water is absorbed.
4. Drain excess water from the pan and stir in almond milk, heating through for 5 minutes.
5. Add the honey and grapefruit.
6. Serve.

Nutrition: *Calories: 231 Fat: 4gCarb: 43g Phosphorus: 165mg Potassium: 370mg Sodium: 135mg*

DARK TURNIP GREENS SMOOTHIE

INGREDIENTS:

- 1 cup of raw turnip greens
- 1 1/2 cup of almond milk
- 1 Tbsp of almond butter
- 1/2 cup of water
- 1/2 tsp of cocoa powder, unsweetened
- 1 Tbsp of dark chocolate chips
- 1/4 tsp of cinnamon
- A pinch of salt
- 1/2 cup of crushed ice

DIRECTIONS:

1. Rinse and clean turnip greens from any dirt.
2. Place the turnip greens in your blender along with all other ingredients.
3. Blend it for 45-60 seconds or until done; smooth and creamy.
4. Serve with or without crushed ice.

Nutrition: *Calories: 131 Carbohydrates: 6g Proteins: 4g Fat: 10g Fiber: 2.5g*

CHERRY BERRY
BULGUR BOWL

INGREDIENTS:

- 1 cup medium-grind bulgur
- 2 cups of water
- Pinch salt
- 1 cup halved and pitted cherries or 1 cup canned cherries, drained
- ½ cup raspberries
- ½ cup blackberries
- 1 tablespoon cherry jam
- 2 cups plain whole-milk yogurt

DIRECTIONS:

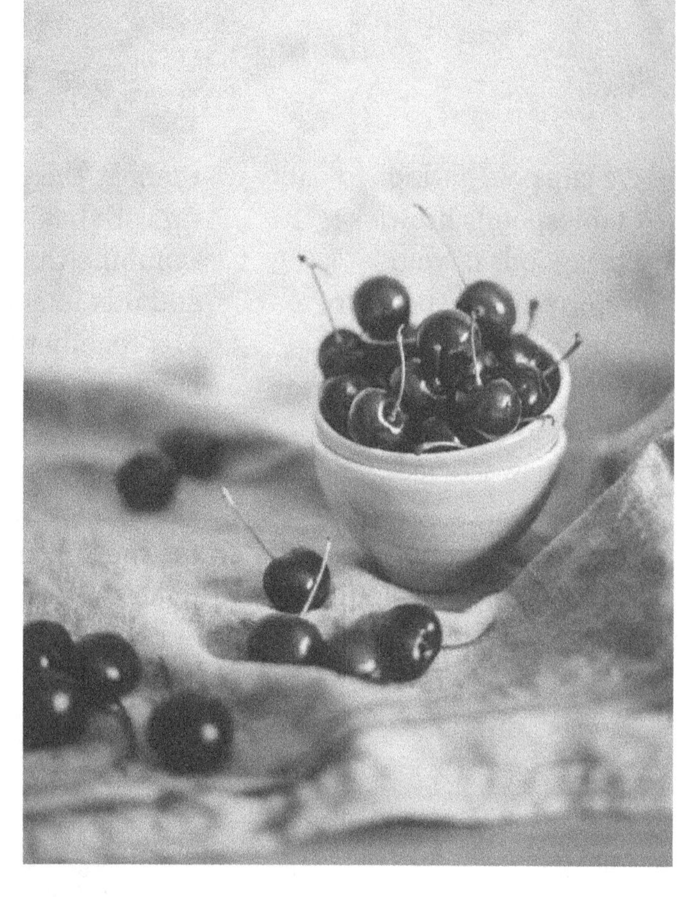

1. Mix the bulgur, water, and salt in a medium saucepan. Do this in medium heat. Bring to a boil.
2. Reduce the heat to low and simmer, partially covered, for 12 to 15 minutes or until the bulgur is almost tender. Cover, and let stand for 5 minutes to finish cooking do this after removing the pan from the heat.
3. While the bulgur is cooking, combine the raspberries and blackberries in a medium bowl. Stir the cherry jam into the fruit.
4. When the bulgur is tender, divide among four bowls. Top each bowl with ½ cup of yogurt and an equal amount of the berry mixture and serve.

Nutrition: *Calories: 242Total fat: 6gSaturated Fat: 3gSodium: 85mgPhosphorus: 237mg Potassium: 438mg Carbohydrates: 44g Fiber: 7g Protein: 9g Sugar: 13g*

BAKED CURRIED APPLE OATMEAL CUPS

INGREDIENTS:

- 3½ cups old-fashioned oats
- 3 tablespoons brown sugar
- 2 teaspoons of your preferred curry powder
- ⅛ teaspoon salt
- 1 cup unsweetened almond milk
- 1 cup unsweetened applesauce
- 1 teaspoon vanilla
- ½ cup chopped walnuts

DIRECTIONS:

1. Preheat the oven to 375°F. Then spray a 12-cup muffin tin with baking spray then set aside.
2. Combine the oats, brown sugar, curry powder, and salt, and mix in a medium bowl.
3. Mix together the milk, applesauce, and vanilla in a small bowl,
4. Stir the liquid ingredients into the dry ingredients and mix until just combined. Stir in the walnuts.
5. Using a scant ⅓ cup for each divide the mixture among the muffin cups.
6. Bake this for 18 to 20 minutes until the oatmeal is firm. Serve.

Nutrition: *For 2 Oatmeal Cups: Calories: 296Total Fat: 10gSaturated Fat: 1gSodium: 84mgPhosphorus: 236mgPotassium: 289mgCarbohydrates: 45gFiber: 6gProtein: 8gSugar: 11g*

CHICKEN EGG ROLLS

INGREDIENTS:

- 1 lb. cooked chicken, diced
- 1/2 lb. bean sprouts
- 1/2 lb. cabbage, shredded
- 1 cup onion, chopped
- 2 tablespoons olive oil
- 1 tablespoon low sodium soy sauce
- 1 garlic clove, minced
- 20 egg roll wrappers
- Oil for frying

DIRECTIONS:

1. Add everything to a suitable bowl except for the roll wrappers.
2. Mix these ingredients well to prepare the filling then marinate for 30 minutes.
3. Place the roll wrappers on the working surface and divide the prepared filling on them.
4. Fold the roll wrappers as per the package instructions and keep them aside.
5. Add oil to a deep wok and heat it to 350 degrees F.
6. Deep the egg rolls until golden brown on all sides.
7. Transfer the egg rolls to a plate lined with a paper towel to absorb all the excess oil.
8. Serve warm.

Nutrition: *Calories: 212 Total Fat: 3.8g Saturated Fat: 0.7g Cholesterol: 29mg Sodium: 29mg Carbohydrate: 29g Dietary Fiber: 1.4g Sugars: 0.9g Protein: 14.9g Calcium: 37mg Phosphorous: 361 mg Potassium: 171mg*

PORK BREAD CASSEROLE

INGREDIENTS:

- 2 tablespoons butter
- 1 lb. pork sausage
- 1 yellow onion, chopped
- 18 slices white bread, cut into cubes
- 2 ½ cups sharp Cheddar cheese, grated
- 1/2 cup fresh parsley, chopped
- 6 large eggs
- 2 cups half-and-half cream
- 1 teaspoon garlic powder
- 1/4 teaspoon black pepper

DIRECTIONS:

1. Switch on your gas oven and preheat it at 325 degrees F.
2. Layer a 9x9 inches casserole dish with bread cubes.
3. Set a suitable-sized skillet over medium-high heat then crumb the sausage in it.
4. Cook the sausage until golden brown, then keep it aside.
5. Blend the eggs with the remaining ingredients in a blender until smooth.
6. Stir in the sausage and spread this mixture over the bread pieces.
7. Bake the bread casserole for 55 minutes approximately in the preheated oven.
8. Slice and serve.
9. Enjoy.

Nutrition: *Calories: 366 Total Fat: 26.4g Saturated Fat: 15.1g Cholesterol: 208mg Sodium: 36mg Carbohydrate: 15.2g Dietary Fiber: 0.9g Sugars: 2.1g Protein: 17.5g Calcium: 378mg Phosphorous: 501mg Potassium: 231mg*

SALMON BAGEL TOAST

INGREDIENTS:

- 1 plain bagel, cut in half
- 2 tablespoons cream cheese
- 1/3 cup English cucumber, thinly sliced
- 3 oz. smoked salmon, sliced
- 3 rings red onion
- 1/2 teaspoon capers, drained

DIRECTIONS:

1. Toast each half of the bagel in a skillet until golden brown.
2. Cover one of the toasted halves with cream cheese.
3. Set the cucumber, salmon, and capers on top of each bagel half.
4. Enjoy.

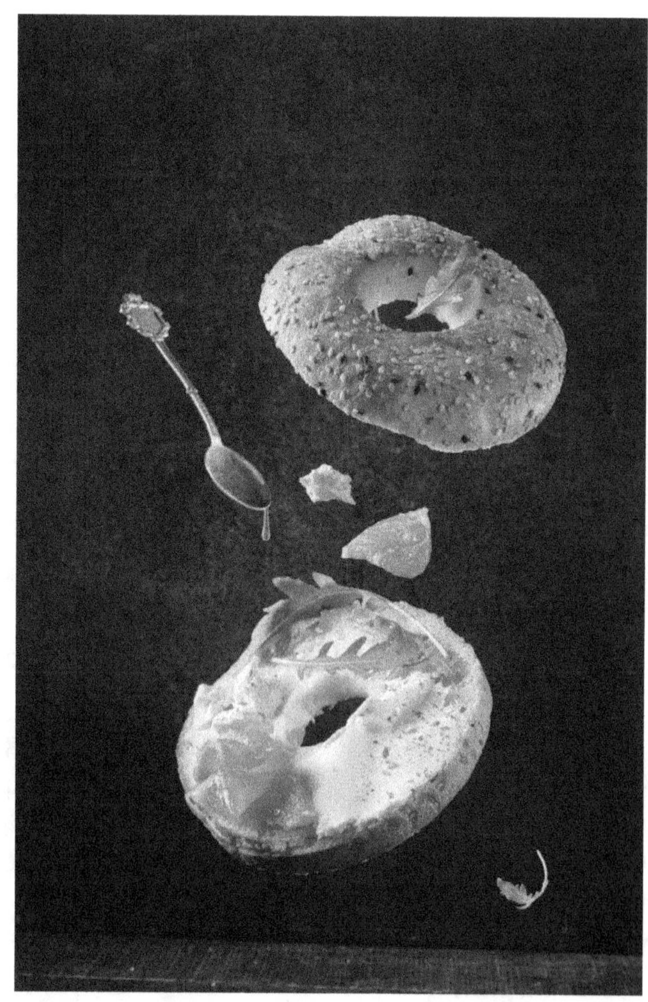

Nutrition: *Calories: 223 Total Fat: .2g Saturated Fat: 2.8g Cholesterol: 21mg Sodium: 1137mg Carbohydrate: 27.5g Dietary Fiber: 1.3g Sugars: 3g Protein: 13.9g Calcium: 62mg Phosphorous: 79mg Potassium: 151mg*

RAW VEGETABLES CHOPPED SALAD

INGREDIENTS:

- Chopped raw veggie salad
- 1 orange pepper (minced) (about 1 cup)
- 1 yellow pepper (small cut) (about 1 cup)
- 5-8 radishes (halve and cut into thin slices) (about 3/4 cup)
- small head of broccoli (minced) (about 2 cups)
- 1 seedless cucumber (small cut) (about 2 cups)
- 1 cup of halved red seedless grapes
- 2-3 tablespoons chopped fresh dill
- 1/4 cup chopped fresh parsley
- 1/4 cup of raw peeled sunflower seeds
- 1/8 cup raw hemp hearts (peeled hemp seeds)
- Oil-free dressing
- Garlic clove (chopped)
- tablespoons of red wine vinegar
- 1 tablespoon of apple cider vinegar
- Juice of 1 lemon
- 1 tablespoon Dijonsenf
- 1 tablespoon pure maple syrup
- 1/2 teaspoon salt (or to taste)
- 1/8 teaspoon pepper (or to taste)

DIRECTIONS:

1. Whisk the ingredients—Chopped raw veggie salad, 1 orange pepper, yellow pepper, radishes, small broccoli head, seedless cucumber, halved red seedless grapes, chopped fresh dill, chopped fresh parsley, raw peeled sunflower seeds, raw hemp hearts, garlic clove, red wine vinegar, apple cider vinegar, lemon, Dijonsenf, pure maple syrup, salt, pepper. For dressing in a small bowl and set aside.
2. Mix all the salad ingredients in a large bowl.
3. Pour the dressing over and wrap well.
4. Cover and then refrigerate it for an hour or two and toss the salad once or twice during this time to coat evenly. Enjoy!

Nutrition: *Calories: 111 Total Fat: 2g Saturated Fat: 1g Cholesterol: 10mg Sodium: 58mg Carbohydrates: 19g Sugar: 18g*

COTTAGE CHEESE PANCAKES

INGREDIENTS:

- 1 cup cottage cheese
- 1/3 cup all-purpose flour
- 2 tablespoons vegetable oil
- 3 eggs, lightly beaten

DIRECTIONS:

1. Begin by beating the eggs in a suitable bowl, then stir in the cottage cheese.
2. Once it is well mixed, stir in the flour.
3. Pour a teaspoon of vegetable oil into a nonstick griddle and heat it.
4. Add ¼ cup of the batter in the griddle and cook for 2 minutes per side until brown.
5. Cook more of the pancakes using the remaining batter.
6. Serve.

Nutrition: *Calories: 196 Total Fat: 11.3g Saturated Fat: 3.1g Cholesterol: 127mg Sodium: 276mg Carbohydrate: 10.3g Dietary Fiber: 0.3g Sugars: 0.5g Protein: 13g Calcium: 58mg Phosphorous: 187 mg Potassium: 110mg*

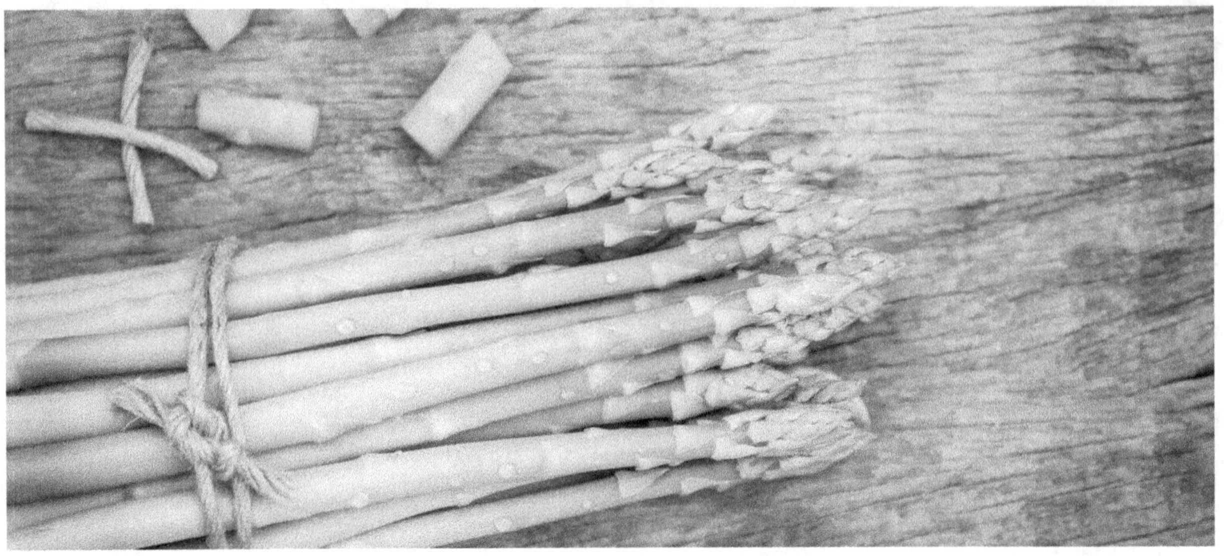

ASPARAGUS BACON HASH

INGREDIENTS:

- 6 slices bacon, diced
- 1/2 onion, chopped
- 2 garlic cloves, sliced
- 2 lb. asparagus, trimmed and chopped
- Black pepper, to taste
- 2 tablespoons Parmesan, grated
- 4 large eggs
- 1/4 teaspoon red pepper flakes

DIRECTIONS:

1. Add the asparagus and a tablespoon of water to a microwave-proof bowl.
2. Cover the veggies and microwave them for 5 minutes until tender.
3. Set a suitable nonstick skillet over moderate heat and layer it with cooking spray.
4. Stir in the onion and sauté for 7 minutes, then toss in the garlic.
5. Stir for 1 minute, then toss in the asparagus, eggs, and red pepper flakes.
6. Reduce the heat to low and cover the vegetables in the pan. Top the eggs with Parmesan cheese.
7. Cook for approximately 15 minutes, then slice to serve.

Nutrition: *Calories: 290 Total Fat: 17.9g Saturated Fat: 6.1g Cholesterol: 220mg Sodium: 256mg Carbohydrate: 11.6g Dietary Fiber: 5.1g Sugars: 5.3g Protein: 23.2g Calcium: 121mg Phosphorous: 247mg Potassium: 715mg*

DARK TURNIP GREENS SMOOTHIE

INGREDIENTS:

- 1 cup of raw turnip greens
- 1 1/2 cup of almond milk
- 1 Tbsp of almond butter
- 1/2 cup of water
- 1/2 tsp of cocoa powder, unsweetened
- 1 Tbsp of dark chocolate chips
- 1/4 tsp of cinnamon
- A pinch of salt
- 1/2 cup of crushed ice

DIRECTIONS:

1. Rinse and clean turnip greens from any dirt.
2. Place the turnip greens in your blender along with all other ingredients.
3. Blend it for 45 - 60 seconds or until done; smooth and creamy.
4. Serve with or without crushed ice.

Nutrition: *Calories: 131 Carbohydrates: 6g Proteins: 4g Fat: 10g Fiber: 2.5g*

BUTTER PECAN AND COCONUT SMOOTHIE

INGREDIENTS:

- 1 cup coconut milk, canned
- 1 scoop Butter Pecan powdered creamer
- 2 cups fresh spinach leaves, chopped
- 1/2 banana frozen or fresh
- 2 Tbsp stevia granulated sweetener to taste
- 1/2 cup water
- 1 cup ice cubes crushed

DIRECTIONS:

1. Place ingredients from the list above in your high-speed blender.
2. Blend for 35-50 seconds or until all ingredients combined well.
3. Add less or more crushed ice.
4. Drink and enjoy!

Nutrition: *Calories: 268 Carbohydrates: 7g Proteins: 6g Fat: 26g Fiber: 1.5g*

FRESH CUCUMBER, KALE AND RASPBERRY SMOOTHIE

INGREDIENTS:

- 1 1/2 cups of cucumber, peeled
- 1/2 cup raw kale leaves
- 1 1/2 cups fresh raspberries
- 1 cup of almond milk
- 1 cup of water
- Ice cubes crushed (optional)
- 2 Tbsp natural sweetener (Stevia, Erythritol...etc.)

DIRECTIONS:

1. Place all ingredients from the list in a food processor or high-speed blender; blend for 35-40 seconds.
2. Serve into chilled glasses.
3. Add more natural sweeter if you like. Enjoy!

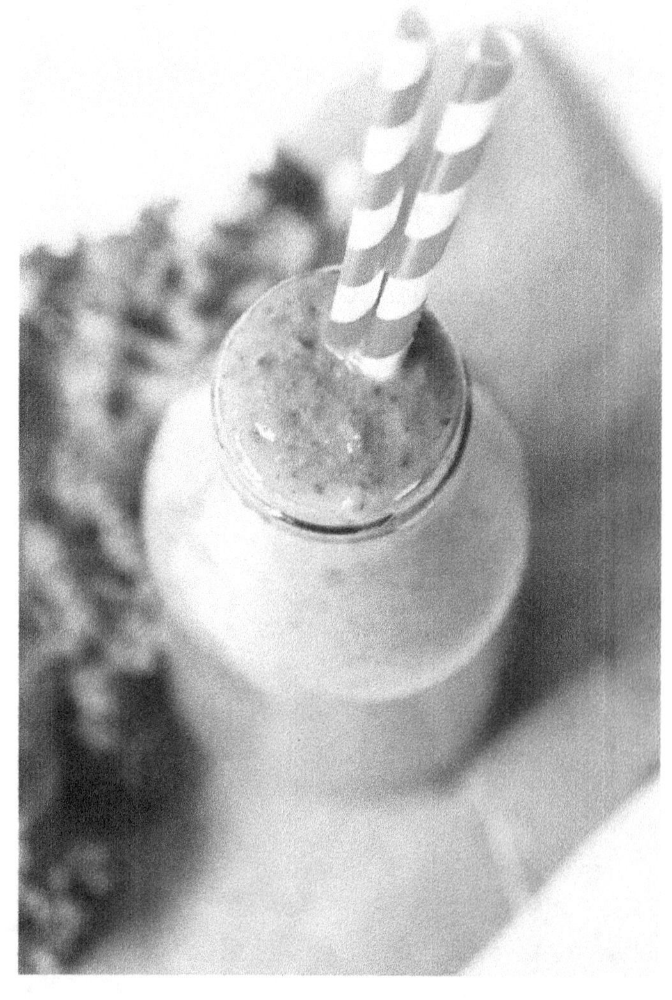

Nutrition: *Calories: 70 Carbohydrates: 8g Proteins: 3g Fat: 6g Fiber: 5g*

FRESH LETTUCE AND CUCUMBER-LEMON SMOOTHIE

INGREDIENTS:

- 2 cups fresh lettuce leaves, chopped (any kind)
- 1 cup of cucumber
- 1 lemon washed and sliced.
- 1/2 avocado
- 2 Tbsp chia seeds
- 1 1/2 cup water or coconut water
- 1/4 cup stevia granulate sweetener (or to taste)

DIRECTIONS:

1. Add all ingredients from the list above into the high-speed blender; blend until completely smooth.
2. Pour your smoothie into chilled glasses and enjoy!

Nutrition: *Calories: 51 Carbohydrates: 4gProteins: 2g Fat: 4g Fiber: 3.5g*

GREEN COCONUT SMOOTHIE

INGREDIENTS:

- 1 1/4 cup coconut milk (canned)
- 2 Tbsp chia seeds
- 1 cup of fresh kale leaves
- 1 cup of spinach leaves
- 1 scoop vanilla protein powder
- 1 cup ice cubes
- Granulated stevia sweetener (to taste; optional)
- 1/2 cup water

DIRECTIONS:

1. Rinse and clean kale and the spinach leaves from any dirt.
2. Add all ingredients into your blender.
3. Blend until you get a nice smoothie.
4. Serve into chilled glass.

Nutrition: *Calories: 179 Carbohydrates: 5g Proteins: 4g Fat: 18g Fiber: 2.5g*

CHEESE SPAGHETTI FRITTATA

INGREDIENTS:

- 4 cups whole-wheat spaghetti, cooked
- 4 teaspoons olive oil
- 3 medium onions, chopped
- 4 large eggs
- ½ cup milk
- ⅓ cup Parmesan cheese, grated
- 2 tablespoons fresh parsley, chopped
- 2 tablespoons fresh basil, chopped
- ½ teaspoon black pepper
- 1 tomato, diced

DIRECTIONS:

1. Set a suitable nonstick skillet over moderate heat and add in the olive oil.
2. Place the spaghetti in the skillet and cook by stirring for 2 minutes on moderate heat.
3. Whisk the eggs with milk, parsley, and black pepper in a bowl.
4. Pour this milky egg mixture over the spaghetti and top it all with basil, cheese, and tomato.
5. Cover the spaghetti frittata again with a lid and cook for approximately 8 minutes on low heat.
6. Slice and serve.

Nutrition: *Calories: 230 Total Fat: 7.8g Saturated Fat: 2g Cholesterol: 127mg Sodium: 77mg Carbohydrate: 31.9g Dietary Fiber: 5.6g Sugars: 4.5g Protein: 11.1g Calcium: 88mg Phosphorous: 368 mg Potassium: 214mg*

PINEAPPLE BREAD

INGREDIENTS:

- 1/3 cup Swerve
- 1/3 cup butter, unsalted
- 2 eggs
- 2 cups flour
- 3 teaspoons baking powder
- 1 cup pineapple, undrained
- 6 cherries, chopped

DIRECTIONS:

1. Whisk the Swerve with the butter in a mixer until fluffy.
2. Stir in the eggs, then beat again.
3. Add the baking powder and flour, then mix well until smooth.
4. Fold in the cherries and pineapple.
5. Spread this cherry-pineapple batter in a 9x5 inch baking pan.
6. Bake the pineapple batter for 1 hour at 350 degrees F.
7. Slice the bread and serve.

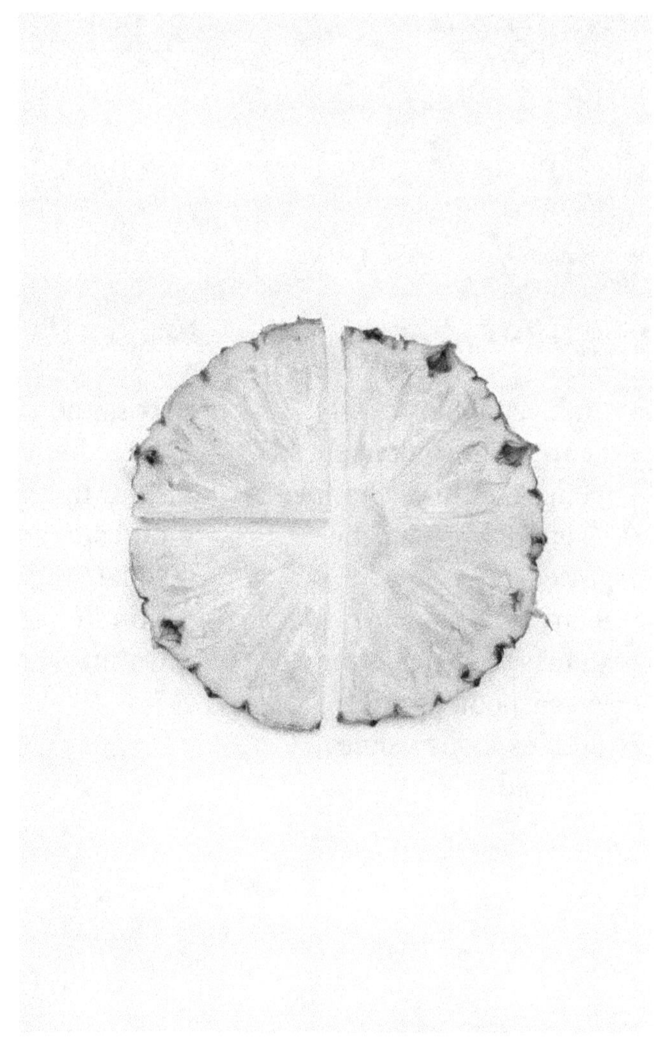

Nutrition: *Calories: 197 Total Fat: 7.2g Saturated Fat: 1.3g Cholesterol: 33mg Sodium: 85mg Carbohydrate: 18.3g Dietary Fiber: 1.1g Sugars: 3g Protein: 4g Calcium: 79mg Phosphorous: 316mg Potassium: 227mg*

PARMESAN ZUCCHINI FRITTATA

INGREDIENTS:

- 1 tablespoon olive oil
- 1 cup yellow onion, sliced
- 3 cups zucchini, chopped
- ½ cup Parmesan cheese, grated
- 8 large eggs
- ½ teaspoon black pepper
- ⅛ teaspoon paprika
- 3 tablespoons parsley, chopped

DIRECTIONS:

1. Toss the zucchinis with the onion, parsley, and all other ingredients in a large bowl.
2. Pour this zucchini-garlic mixture into an 11x7 inches pan and spread it evenly.
3. Bake the zucchini casserole for approximately 35 minutes at 350 degrees F.
4. Cut in slices and serve.

Nutrition: *Calories: 142 Total Fat: 9.7g Saturated Fat: 2.8g Cholesterol: 250mg Sodium: 123mg Carbohydrate: 4.7g Dietary Fiber: 1.3g Sugars: 2.4g Protein: 10.2g Calcium: 73mg Phosphorous: 375mg Potassium: 286mg*

TEXAS TOAST
CASSEROLE

INGREDIENTS:

- 1/2 cup butter, melted
- 1 cup brown Swerve
- 1 lb. Texas Toast bread, sliced
- 4 large eggs
- 1 1/2 cup milk
- 1 tablespoon vanilla extract
- 2 tablespoons Swerve
- 2 teaspoons cinnamon
- Maple syrup for serving

DIRECTIONS:

1. Layer a 9x13 inches baking pan with cooking spray.
2. Spread the bread slices at the bottom of the prepared pan.
3. Whisk the eggs with the remaining ingredients in a mixer.
4. Pour this mixture over the bread slices evenly.
5. Bake the bread for 30 minutes at 350 degrees F in a preheated oven.
6. Serve.

Nutrition: *Calories: 332 Total Fat: 13.7g Saturated Fat: 6.9g Cholesterol: 102mg Sodium: 350mg Carbohydrate: 22.6g Dietary Fiber: 2g Sugars: 6g Protein: 7.4g Calcium: 143mg Phosphorous: 186mg Potassium: 74mg*

GARLIC MAYO BREAD

INGREDIENTS:

- 3 tablespoons vegetable oil
- 4 cloves garlic, minced
- 2 teaspoons paprika
- Dash cayenne pepper
- 1 teaspoon lemon juice
- 2 tablespoons Parmesan cheese, grated
- 3/4 cup mayonnaise
- 1 loaf (1 lb.) French bread, sliced
- 1 teaspoon Italian herbs

DIRECTIONS:

1. Mix the garlic with the oil in a small bowl and leave it overnight.
2. Discard the garlic from the bowl and keep the garlic-infused oil.
3. Mix the garlic-oil with cayenne, paprika, lemon juice, mayonnaise, and Parmesan.
4. Place the bread slices in a baking tray lined with parchment paper.
5. Top these slices with the mayonnaise mixture and drizzle the Italian herbs on top.
6. Broil these slices for 5 minutes until golden brown.
7. Serve warm.

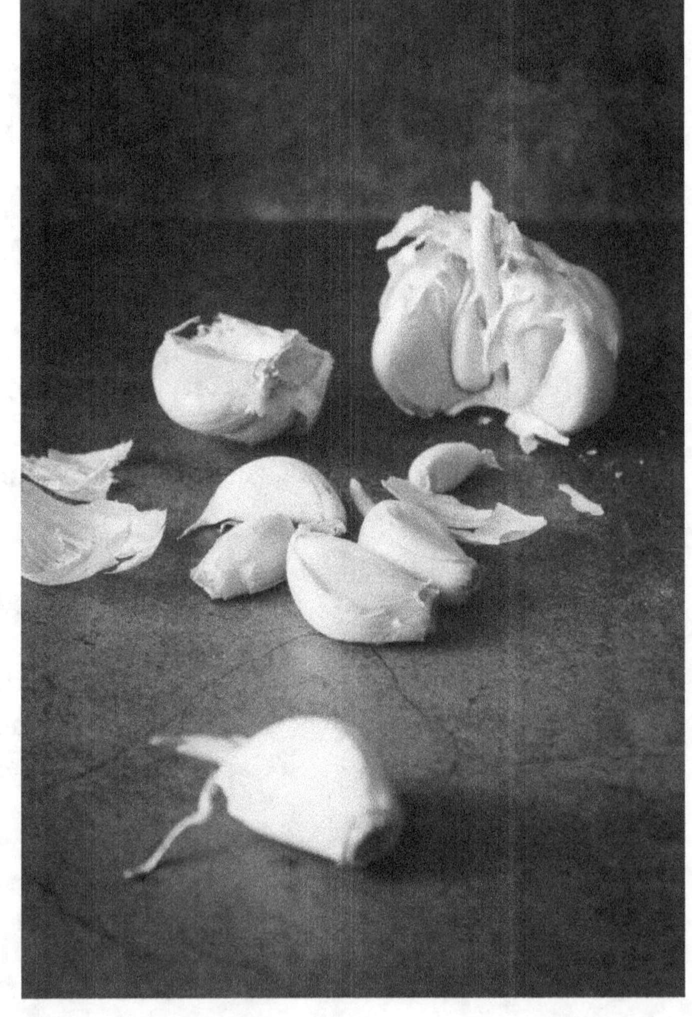

Nutrition: *Calories: 217 Total Fat: 7.9g Saturated Fat: 1.8g Cholesterol: 5mg Sodium: 423mg Carbohydrate: 30.3g Dietary Fiber: 1.3g Sugars: 2g Protein: 7g Calcium: 56mg Phosphorous: 347mg Potassium: 72mg*

STRAWBERRY

TOPPED WAFFLES

INGREDIENTS:

- 1 cup flour
- 1/4 cup Swerve
- 1 ¾ teaspoons baking powder
- 1 egg, separated
- ¾ cup milk
- ½ cup butter, melted
- ½ teaspoon vanilla extract
- Fresh strawberries, sliced

DIRECTIONS:

1. Prepare and preheat your waffle pan following the instructions of the machine.
2. Begin by mixing the flour with Swerve and baking soda in a bowl.
3. Separate the egg yolks from the egg whites, keeping them in two separate bowls.
4. Add the milk and vanilla extract to the egg yolks.
5. Stir the melted butter and mix well until smooth.
6. Now beat the egg whites with an electric beater until foamy and fluffy.
7. Fold this fluffy composition in the egg yolk mixture.
8. Mix it gently until smooth, then add in the flour mixture.
9. Stir again to make a smooth mixture.
10. Pour a half cup of the waffle batter into a preheated pan and cook until the waffle is done.
11. Cook more waffles with the remaining batter.
12. Serve fresh with strawberries on top.

Nutrition: *Calories: 342 Total Fat: 20.5g Saturated Fat: 12.5g Cholesterol: 88mg Sodium: 156mg Carbohydrate: 21g Dietary Fiber: 0.7g Sugars: 3.5g Protein: 4.8g Calcium: 107mg Phosphorous: 126mg Potassium: 233mg*

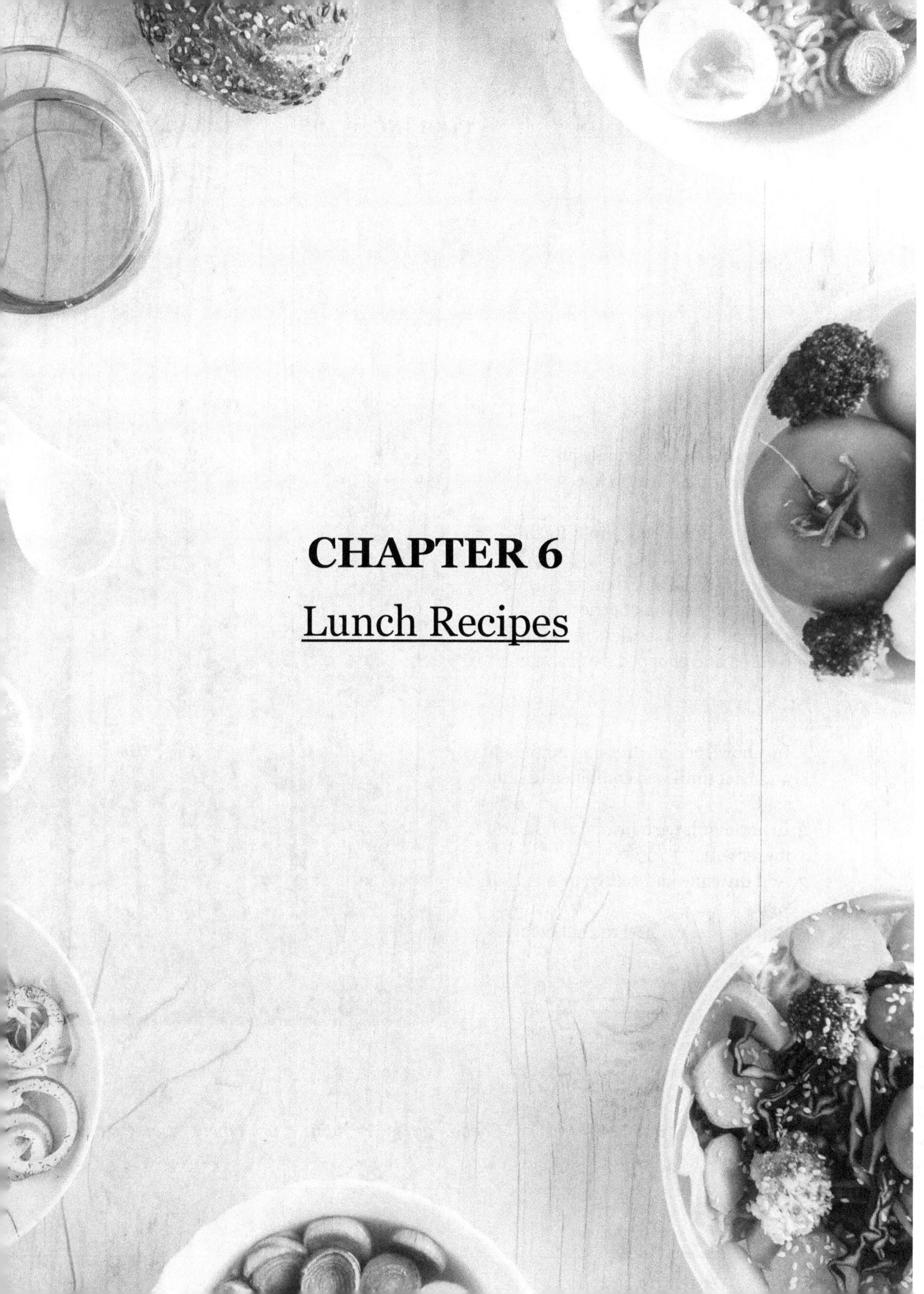

CHAPTER 6

<u>Lunch Recipes</u>

ENERGETIC
FRUITY SALAD

INGREDIENTS:

- ½ cup of fresh pineapple juice
- 2 tbsp. of fresh lemon juice
- For Salad:
- 2 cups of hulled and sliced fresh strawberries
- 2 cups of fresh blackberries
- 2 cups of fresh blueberries
- 1 cup of halved seedless red grapes
- 6 cored and chopped fresh apples

DIRECTIONS:

1. In a bowl, add all dressing ingredients and beat until well combined. Keep aside.
2. In another large bowl, mix all salad ingredients.
3. Add dressing and gently, toss to coat well.
4. Refrigerate, covered to chill before serving.

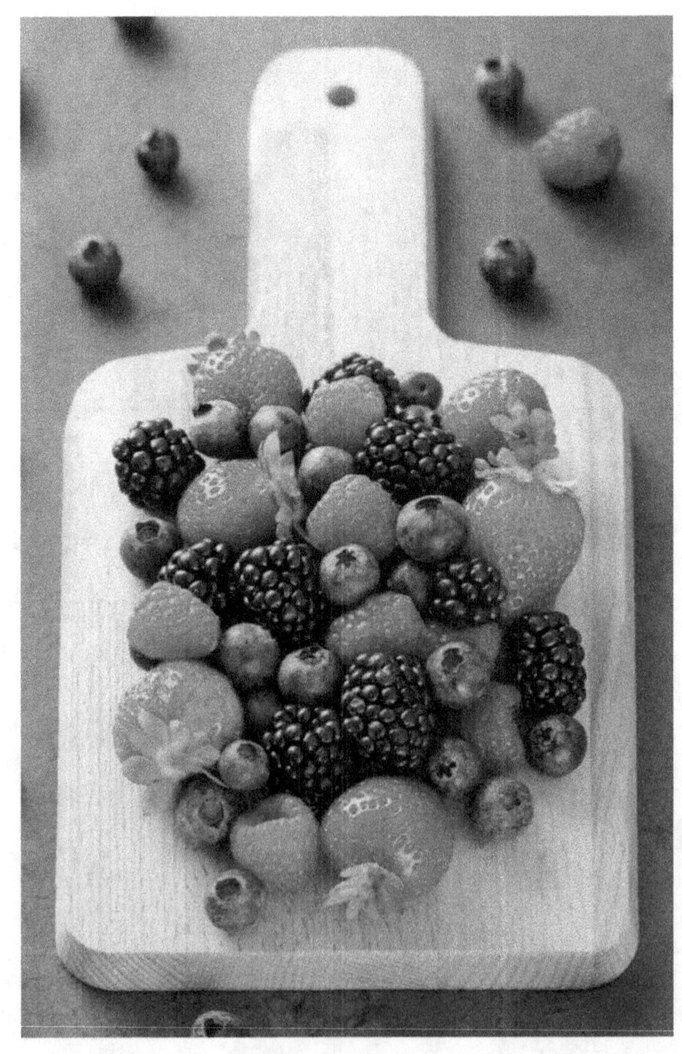

Nutrition:*Calories: 116Fat: 0.5g Carbs: 29.3g Protein: 1.2g Fiber: 5.3g Potassium: 276mg Sodium: 3mg*

APPEALING

GREEN SALAD

INGREDIENTS:

- 1 tbsp. of shallot, minced
- 1/3 cup of olive oil
- 2 tbsp. of fresh lemon juice
- 1 tsp. of honey
- Freshly ground black pepper, to taste

For Salad:

- 1½ cups of chopped broccoli florets
- 1½ cups of shredded cabbage
- 4 cups of chopped lettuce

DIRECTIONS:

1. In a bowl, add all dressing ingredients and beat until well combined. Keep aside. In another large bowl, mix all salad ingredients.
2. Add dressing and gently, toss to coat well. Serve immediately.

Nutrition: *Calories: 179Fat: 17.1g Carbs: 7.5g Protein: 1.7g Fiber: 1.9g Potassium: 249mg Sodium: 21mg*

EXCELLENT VEGGIE SANDWICHES

INGREDIENTS:

- 1 large sliced tomato
- ½ of sliced cucumber
- ½ cup of thinly sliced red onion
- 1 cup of chopped romaine lettuce leaves
- ½ cup of low-sodium mayonnaise
- 8 toasted white bread slices

DIRECTIONS:

1. In a large bowl, mix together tomato, cucumber, onion and lettuce. Spread mayonnaise over each slice evenly.
2. Divide tomato mixture over 4 slices evenly. Cover with remaining slices.
3. With a knife, carefully cut the sandwiches diagonally and serve.

Nutrition: *Calories: 92 Fat: 5.3g Carbs: 10.5g Protein: 1.2g Fiber: 0.8g Potassium: 112mg Sodium: 168mg*

LUNCHTIME
STAPLE SANDWICHES

INGREDIENTS:

- 3 tsp. of low-sodium mayonnaise
- 2 toasted white bread slices
- 3 tbsp. of chopped unsalted cooked turkey
- 2 thin apple slices
- 2 tbsp. of low-fat cheddar cheese
- 1 tsp. of olive oil

DIRECTIONS:

1. Spread mayonnaise over each slice evenly.
2. Place turkey over 1 slice, followed by apple slices and cheese.
3. Cover with the remaining slice to make a sandwich.
4. Grease a large non-stick frying pan with oil and heat on medium heat.
5. Place the sandwich in a frying pan and with the back of a spoon, gently, press down.
6. Cook for about 1-2 minutes.
7. Carefully, flip the whole sandwich and cook for about 1-2 minutes.
8. Transfer the sandwich to a serving plate.
9. With a knife, carefully cut the sandwich diagonally and serve.

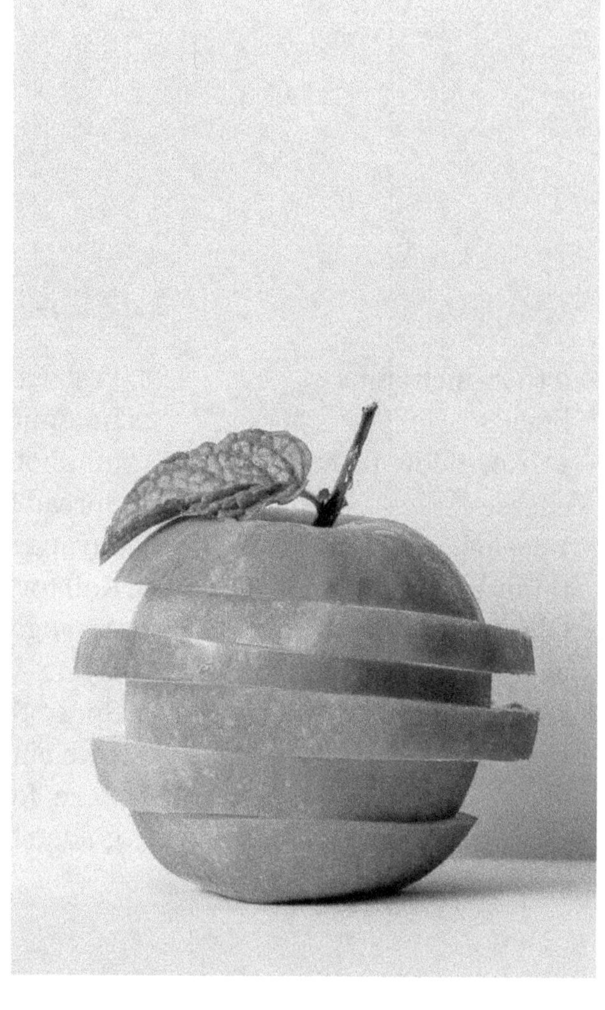

Nutrition: *Calories: 239 Fat: 8.5g Carbs: 37.2g Protein: 7g Fiber: 5.6g Potassium: 294mg Sodium: 169mg*

GREEK STYLE
PITA ROLLS

INGREDIENTS:

- 2 (6½-inch) pita breads
- 1 tbsp. of low-fat cream cheese
- 1 peeled, cored and thinly sliced apple
- Olive oil cooking spray, as required
- 1/8 tsp. of ground cinnamon

DIRECTIONS:

1. Preheat the oven to 400 degrees F.
2. In a microwave safe plate, place tortillas and microwave for about 10 seconds to soften.
3. Spread the cream cheese over each tortilla evenly.
4. Arrange apple slices in the center of each tortilla evenly.
5. Roll tortillas to secure the filling.
6. Arrange the tortilla rolls onto a baking sheet in a single layer.
7. Spray the rolls with cooking spray evenly and sprinkle with cinnamon.
8. Bake for about 10 minutes or until the top becomes golden brown.

Nutrition:_Calories: 129Fat: 2.2g Carbs: 24.6g Protein: 3.3g Fiber: 2.1g Potassium: 102mg Sodium: 176mg_

HEALTHIER PITA VEGGIE ROLLS

INGREDIENTS:

- 1 cup of shredded romaine lettuce
- 1 seeded and chopped red bell pepper
- ½ cup of chopped cucumber
- 1 small seeded and chopped tomato
- 1 small chopped red onion
- 1 finely minced garlic clove
- 1 tbsp. of olive oil
- ½ tbsp. of fresh lemon juice
- Freshly ground black pepper, to taste
- 3 (6½-inch) pita breads

DIRECTIONS:

1. In a large bowl, add all ingredients except pita breads and gently toss to coat well.
2. Arrange pita breads onto serving plates.
3. Place veggie mixture in the center of each pita bread evenly. Roll the pita bread and serve.

Nutrition: *Calories: 120Fat: 2.8g Carbs: 20.7g Protein: 3.3g Fiber: 1.5g Potassium: 156mg Sodium: 164mg*

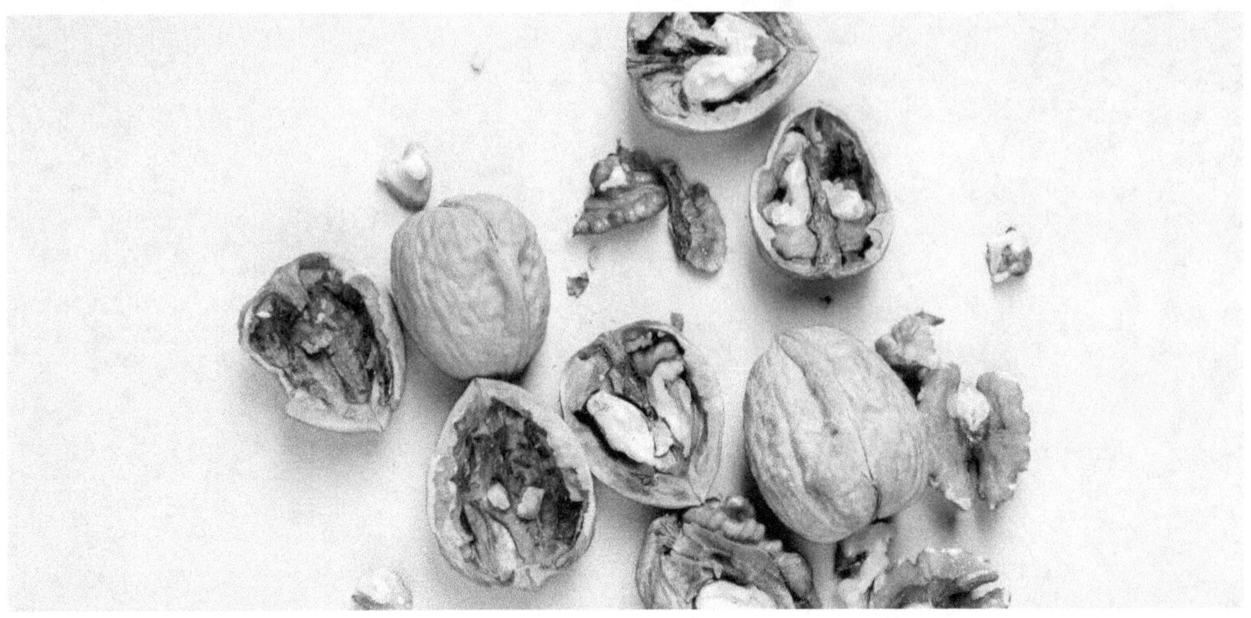

CRUNCHY VEGGIE WRAPS

INGREDIENTS:

- ¾ cup of shredded purple cabbage
- ¾ cup of shredded green cabbage
- ½ cup of peeled and julienned cucumber
- ½ cup of peeled and julienned carrot
- ¼ cup of chopped walnuts
- 2 tbsp. of olive oil
- 1 tbsp. of fresh lemon juice
- Pinch of salt
- Freshly ground black pepper, to taste
- 6 medium butter lettuce leaves

DIRECTIONS:

1. In a large bowl, add all ingredients except lettuce and toss to coat well.
2. Place the lettuce leaves onto serving plates.
3. Divide the veggie mixture over each leaf evenly. Top with tofu sauce and serve.

Nutrition: *Calories: 42Fat: 3.1g Carbs: 2.9g Protein: 1.6g Fiber: 1.1g Potassium: 106mg Sodium: 10mg*

SAUCY FISH DILL

INGREDIENTS:

- 4 (4 oz.) salmon fillets

Dill Sauce:

- 1 cup whipped cream cheese
- 4 minced garlic cloves
- ½ small onion, diced
- 3 tablespoons fresh or dried dill (as desired)
- ½ teaspoon ground pepper
- 1 teaspoon Mrs. Dash (optional)
- 2 drops of hot sauce (optional)

DIRECTIONS:

1. Place the salmon fillets in a moderately shallow baking stray.
2. Whisk the cream cheese and all the dill-sauce ingredients in a bowl.
3. Spread the dill-sauce over the fillets liberally.
4. Cover the fillet pan with a foil sheet and bake for 15 minutes at 350 degrees F.
5. Serve warm.

Nutrition: *Calories: 432 Total Fat: 26.7g Saturated Fat: 12.9g Cholesterol: 42mg Sodium: 280mg Carbohydrate: 5g Dietary Fiber: 0.9g Sugars: 2.25g Protein: 35.8g Calcium: 141mg Phosphorous: 265mg Potassium: 590mg*

LEMON PEPPER

TROUT

INGREDIENTS:

- 1 lb. trout fillets
- 1 lb. asparagus
- 3 tablespoons olive oil
- 5 garlic cloves, minced
- 1/2 teaspoon black pepper
- 1/2 lemon, sliced

DIRECTIONS:

1. Prepare and preheat the gas oven at 350 degrees F.
2. Rub the washed and dried fillets with oil then place them in a baking tray.
3. Top the fish with lemon slices, black pepper, and garlic cloves.
4. Spread the asparagus around the fish.
5. Bake the fish for 15 minutes approximately in the preheated oven.
6. Serve warm.

Nutrition:*Calories: 336 Total Fat: 20.3g Saturated Fat: 3.2g Cholesterol: 84mg Sodium: 370mg Carbohydrate: 6.5g Dietary Fiber: 2.7g Sugars: 2.4g Protein: 33g Calcium: 100mg Phosphorous: 107mg Potassium: 383mg*

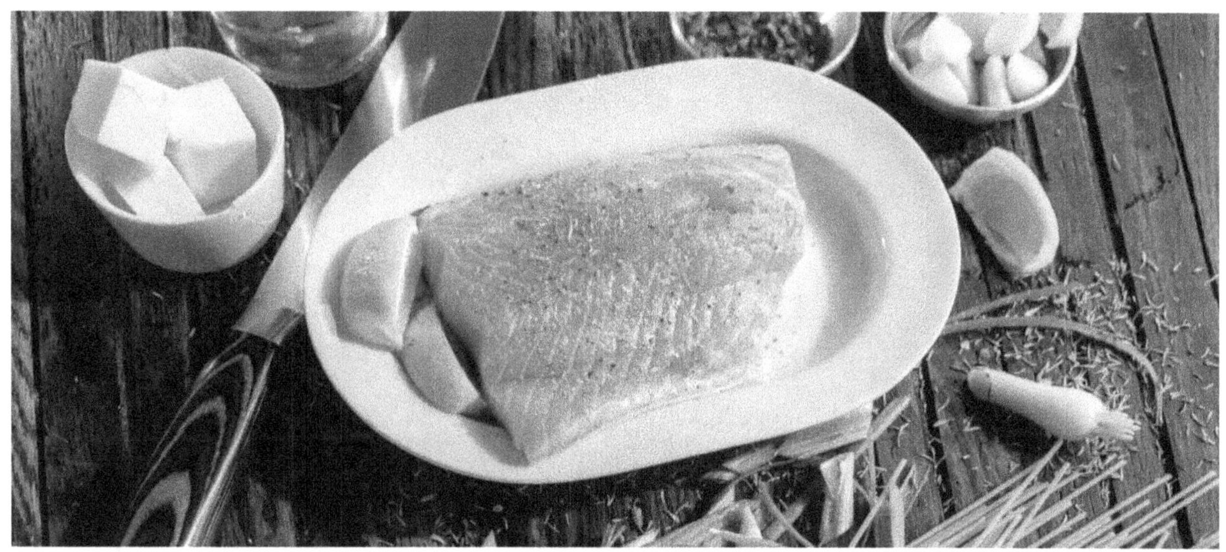

HERBED VEGETABLE TROUT

INGREDIENTS:

- 14 oz. trout fillets
- 1/2 teaspoon herb seasoning blend
- 1 lemon, sliced
- 2 green onions, sliced
- 1 stalk celery, chopped
- 1 medium carrot, julienne

DIRECTIONS:

1. Prepare and preheat a charcoal grill over moderate heat.
2. Place the trout fillets over a large piece of foil and drizzle herb seasoning on top.
3. Spread the lemon slices, carrots, celery, and green onions over the fish.
4. Cover the fish with foil and pack it.
5. Place the packed fish in the grill and cook for 15 minutes.
6. Once done, remove the foil from the fish.
7. Serve.

Nutrition: *Calories: 202 Total Fat: 8.5g Saturated Fat: 1.5g Cholesterol: 73mg Sodium: 82mg Carbohydrate: 3.5g Dietary Fiber: 1.1g Sugars: 1.3g Protein: 26.9g Calcium: 70mg Phosphorous: 287mg Potassium: 560mg*

CITRUS GLAZED

SALMON

INGREDIENTS:

- 2 garlic cloves, crushed
- 1 1/2 tablespoons lemon juice
- 2 tablespoons olive oil
- 1 tablespoon butter
- 1 tablespoon Dijon mustard
- 2 dashes cayenne pepper
- 1 teaspoon dried basil leaves
- 1 teaspoon dried dill
- 24 oz. salmon filet

DIRECTIONS:

1. Place a 1-quart saucepan over moderate heat and add the oil, butter, garlic, lemon juice, mustard, cayenne pepper, dill, and basil to the pan.
2. Stir this mixture for 5 minutes after it has boiled.
3. Prepare and preheat a charcoal grill over moderate heat.
4. Place the fish on a foil sheet and fold the edges to make a foil tray.
5. Pour the prepared sauce over the fish.
6. Place the fish in the foil in the preheated grill and cook for 12 minutes.
7. Slice and serve.

Nutrition: *Calories: 401 Total Fat: 20.5g Saturated Fat: 5.3g Cholesterol: 144mg Sodium: 256mg Carbohydrate: 0.5g Dietary Fiber: 0.2g Sugars: 0.1g Protein: 48.4g Calcium: 549mg Phosphorous: 214mg Potassium: 446mg*

BROILED SALMON

FILLETS

INGREDIENTS:

- 1 tablespoon ginger root, grated
- 1 clove garlic, minced
- ¼ cup maple syrup
- 1 tablespoon hot pepper sauce
- 4 salmon fillets, skinless

DIRECTIONS:

1. Grease a pan with cooking spray and place it over moderate heat.
2. Add the ginger and garlic and sauté for 3 minutes then transfer to a bowl.
3. Add the hot pepper sauce and maple syrup to the ginger-garlic.
4. Mix well and keep this mixture aside.
5. Place the salmon fillet in a suitable baking tray, greased with cooking oil.
6. Brush the maple sauce over the fillets liberally
7. Broil them for 10 minutes in the oven at broiler settings.
8. Serve warm.

Nutrition:*Calories: 289 Total Fat: 11.1g Saturated Fat: 1.6g Cholesterol: 78mg Sodium: 80mg Carbohydrate: 13.6g Dietary Fiber: 0g Sugars: 11.8g Protein: 34.6g Calcium: 78mg Phosphorous: 230mg Potassium: 331mg*

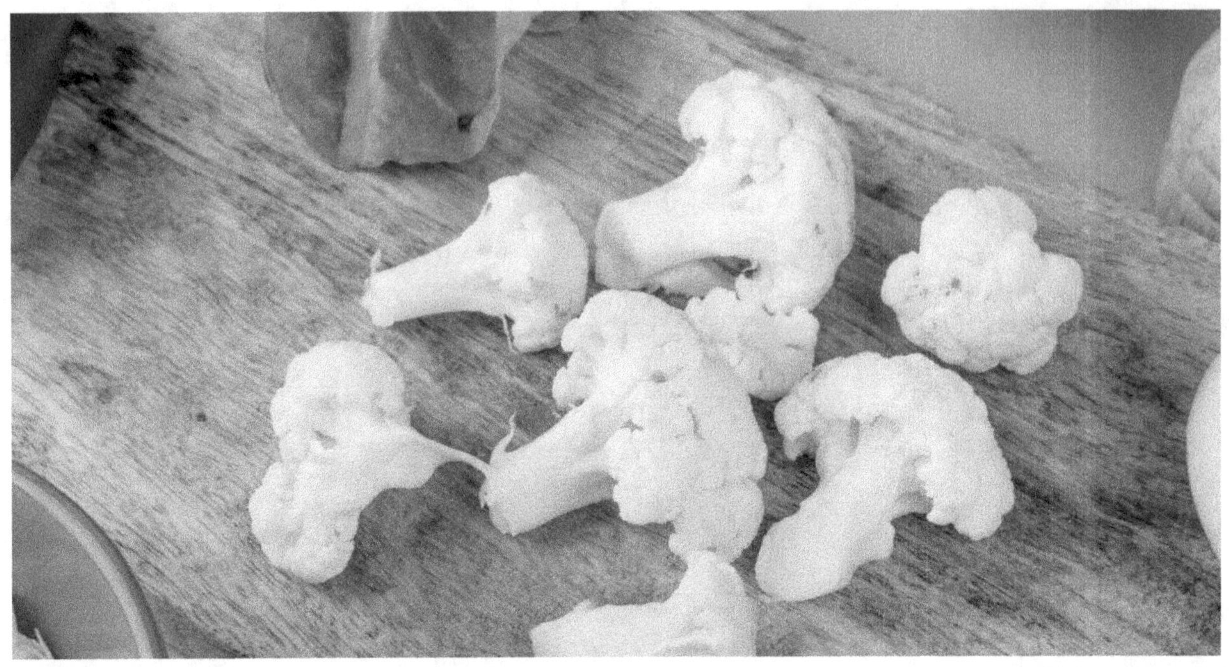

TANTALIZING CAULIFLOWER
AND DILL MASH

INGREDIENTS:

- 1 cauliflower head, florets separated
- 1/3 cup dill, chopped
- 6 garlic cloves
- 2 tablespoons olive oil
- Pinch of black pepper

DIRECTIONS:

1. Add cauliflower to Slow Cooker.
2. Add dill, garlic and water to cover them.
3. Place lid and cook on HIGH for 5 hours.
4. Drain the flowers.
5. Season with pepper and add oil, mash using potato masher.
6. Whisk and serve.
7. Enjoy!

Nutrition: *Calories: 207 Fat: 4g Carbohydrates: 14g Protein: 3g*

BROILED SHRIMP

INGREDIENTS:

- 1 lb. shrimp in shell
- 1/2 cup unsalted butter, melted
- 2 teaspoons lemon juice
- 2 tablespoons chopped onion
- 1 clove garlic, minced
- 1/8 teaspoon pepper

DIRECTIONS:

1. Toss the shrimp with the butter, lemon juice, onion, garlic, and pepper in a bowl.
2. Spread the seasoned shrimp in a baking tray.
3. Broil for 5 minutes in an oven on broiler setting.
4. Serve warm.

Nutrition: *Calories: 164 Total Fat: 12.8g Saturated Fat: 7.4g Cholesterol: 167mg Sodium: 242mg Carbohydrate: 0.6g Dietary Fiber: 0.1g Sugars: 0.2g Protein: 14.6g Calcium: 45mg Phosphorous: 215mg Potassium: 228mg*

GRILLED LEMONY COD

INGREDIENTS:

- 1 lb. cod fillets
- 1 teaspoon salt-free lemon pepper seasoning
- 1/4 cup lemon juice

DIRECTIONS:

1. Rub the cod fillets with lemon pepper seasoning and lemon juice.
2. Grease a baking tray with cooking spray and place the salmon in the baking tray.
3. Bake the fish for 10 minutes at 350 degrees F in a preheated oven.
4. Serve warm.

Nutrition: *Calories: 155 Total Fat: 7.1g Saturated Fat: 1.1g Cholesterol: 50mg Sodium: 53mg Carbohydrate: 0.7g Dietary Fiber: 0.2g Sugars: 0.3g Protein: 22.2g Calcium: 43mg Phosphorous: 237mg Potassium: 461mg*

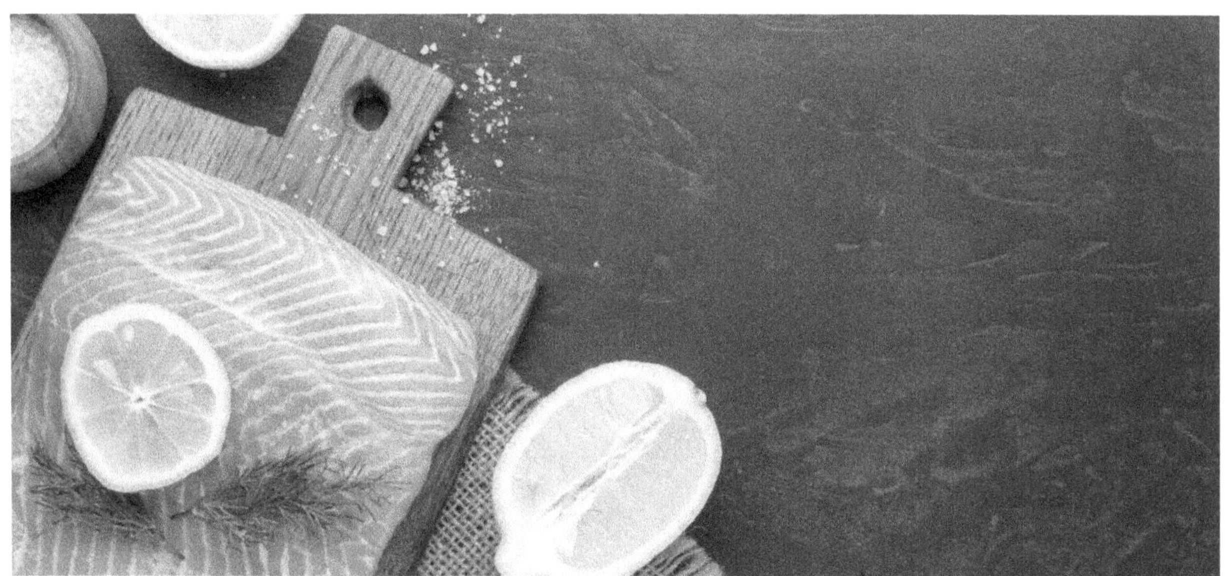

SPICED HONEY SALMON

INGREDIENTS:

- 3 tablespoons honey
- 3/4 teaspoon lemon peel
- 1/2 teaspoon black pepper
- 1/2 teaspoon garlic powder
- 1 teaspoon water
- 16 oz. salmon fillets
- 2 tablespoons olive oil
- Dill, chopped, to serve

DIRECTIONS:

1. Whisk the lemon peel with honey, garlic powder, hot water, and ground pepper in a small bowl.
2. Rub this honey mixture over the salmon fillet liberally.
3. Set a suitable skillet over moderate heat and add olive oil to heat.
4. Set the spiced salmon fillets in the pan and sear them for 4 minutes per side.
5. Garnish with dill.
6. Serve warm.

Nutrition: *Calories: 264 Total Fat: 14.1g Saturated Fat: 2g Cholesterol: 50mg Sodium: 55mg Carbohydrate: 14g Dietary Fiber: 0.4g Sugars: 13.4g Protein: 22.5g Calcium: 67mg Phosphorous: 174mg Potassium: 507mg*

SURPRISINGLY TASTY
CHICKEN WRAPS

INGREDIENTS:

- 4-ounce of cut into strips unsalted cooked chicken breast
- ½ cup of hulled and thinly sliced fresh strawberries
- 1 thinly sliced English cucumber
- 1 tbsp. of chopped fresh mint leaves
- 4 large lettuce leaves

DIRECTIONS:

1. In a large bowl, add all ingredients except lettuce leaves and gently toss to coat well.
2. Place the lettuce leaves onto serving plates.
3. Divide the chicken mixture over each leaf evenly.
4. Serve immediately.

Nutrition: *Calories: 74Fat: 2.3g Carbs: 4.7g Protein: 8.9g Potassium: 235mg Sodium: 27mg*

DELICIOUS VEGETARIAN LASAGNA

INGREDIENTS:

- 1 teaspoon basil
- 1 tablespoon olive oil
- ½ sliced red pepper
- 3 lasagna sheets
- ½ diced red onion
- ¼ teaspoon black pepper
- 1 cup rice milk
- 1 minced garlic clove
- 1 cup sliced eggplant
- ½ sliced zucchini
- ½ pack soft tofu
- 1 teaspoon oregano

DIRECTIONS:

1. Preheat oven to 325°F/Gas Mark 3. Slice zucchini, eggplant and pepper into vertical strips.
2. Add the rice milk and tofu to a food processor and blitz until smooth. Set aside.
3. Heat the oil in a skillet over medium heat and add the onions and garlic for 3-4 minutes or until soft.
4. Sprinkle in the herbs and pepper and allow to stir through for 5-6 minutes until hot.
5. Into a lasagna or suitable oven dish, layer 1 lasagna sheet, then 1/3 the eggplant, followed by 1/3 zucchini, then 1/3 pepper before pouring over 1/3 of tofu white sauce.
6. Repeat for the next 2 layers, finishing with the white sauce.
7. Add to the oven for 40-50 minutes or until veg is soft and can easily be sliced into servings.

Nutrition: *Calories: 235Protein: 5 gCarbs: 10gFat: 9gSodium: 35mgPotassium: 129mg Phosphorus: 66mg*

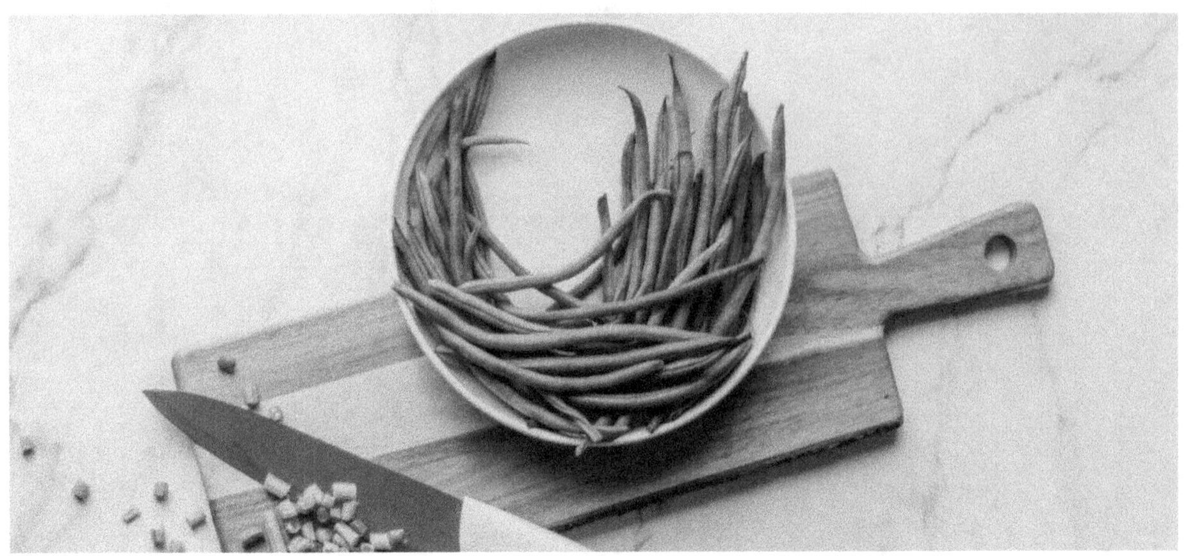

CHILI TOFU NOODLES

INGREDIENTS:

- ½ diced red chili
- 2 cups rice noodles
- ½ juiced lime
- 6 ounce pressed and cubed silken firm tofu
- 1 teaspoon grated fresh ginger
- 1 tablespoon coconut oil
- 1 cup green beans
- 1 minced garlic clove

DIRECTIONS:

1. Steam the green beans for 10-12 minutes or according to package directions and drain.
2. Cook the noodles in a pot of boiling water for 10-15 minutes or according to package directions.
3. Meanwhile, heat a wok or skillet on a high heat and add coconut oil.
4. Now add the tofu, chili flakes, garlic, and ginger and sauté for 5-10 minutes.
5. After doing that, drain in the noodles along with the green beans and lime juice, then add it to the wok.
6. Toss to coat.
7. Serve hot!

Nutrition: *Calories: 246 Protein: 10g Carbs: 28g Fat: 12g Sodium: 25mg Potassium: 126mg Phosphorus: 79mg*

CURRIED CAULIFLOWER

INGREDIENTS:

- 1 teaspoon turmeric
- 1 diced onion
- 1 tablespoon chopped fresh cilantro
- 1 teaspoon cumin
- ½ diced chili
- ½ cup water
- 1 minced garlic clove
- 1 tablespoon coconut oil
- 1 teaspoon garam masala
- 2 cups cauliflower florets

DIRECTIONS:

1. Add the oil to a skillet on medium heat.
2. Sauté the onion and garlic for 5 minutes until soft.
3. Add in the cumin, turmeric and garam masala and stir to release the aromas.
4. Now add the chili to the pan along with the cauliflower.
5. Stir to coat.
6. Pour in the water and reduce the heat to a simmer for 15 minutes.
7. Garnish with cilantro to serve.

Nutrition: *Calories 108 Protein: 2g Carbs: 11g Fat: 7g Sodium: 35mg Potassium: 328mg Phosphorus: 39mg*

ELEGANT VEGGIE

TORTILLAS

INGREDIENTS:

- 1½ cups of chopped broccoli florets
- 1½ cups of chopped cauliflower florets
- 1 tablespoon of water
- 2 teaspoon of canola oil
- 1½ cups of chopped onion
- 1 minced garlic clove
- 2 tablespoons of finely chopped fresh parsley
- 1 cup of low-cholesterol liquid egg substitute
- Freshly ground black pepper, to taste
- 4 (6-ounce) warmed corn tortillas

DIRECTIONS:

1. In a microwave bowl, place broccoli, cauliflower and water and microwave, covered for about 3-5 minutes.
2. Remove from microwave and drain any liquid.
3. Heat oil on medium heat.
4. Add onion and sauté for about 4-5 minutes.
5. Add garlic and then sauté it for about 1 minute.
6. Stir in broccoli, cauliflower, parsley, egg substitute and black pepper.
7. Reduce the heat and let it simmer for about 10 minutes.
8. Remove from heat and keep aside to cool slightly.
9. Place broccoli mixture over ¼ of each tortilla.
10. Fold the outside edges inward and roll up like a burrito.
11. Secure each tortilla with toothpicks to secure the filling.
12. Cut each tortilla in half and serve.

Nutrition: *Calories: 217 Fat: 3.3g Carbs: 41g Protein: 8.1g Fiber: 6.3g Potassium: 289mg Sodium: 87mg*

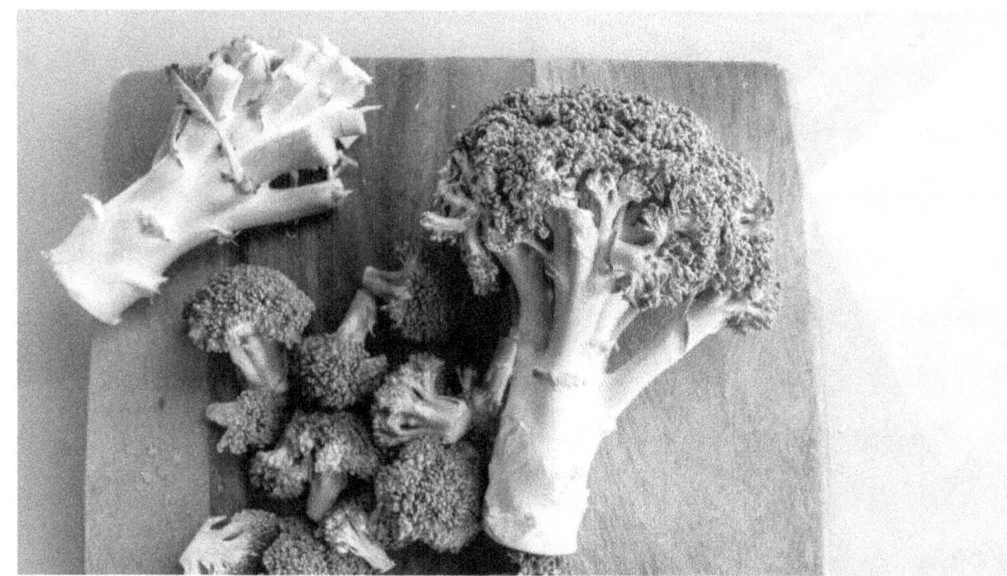

SIMPLE BROCCOLI STIR-FRY

INGREDIENTS:

- 1 tablespoon of olive oil
- 1 minced garlic clove
- 2 cups of broccoli florets
- 2 tablespoons of water

DIRECTIONS:

1. Heat oil on medium heat.
2. Add garlic and then sauté for about 1 minute.
3. Add the broccoli and stir fry for about 2 minutes.
4. Stir in water and stir fry for about 4-5 minutes.
5. Serve warm.

Nutrition:_Calories: 4 Fat: 3.6g Carbs: 3.3g Protein: 1.3g Fiber: 1.2g Potassium: 147mg Sodium: 15mg_

BRAISED CABBAGE

INGREDIENTS:

- 1½ teaspoon of olive oil
- 2 minced garlic cloves
- 1 thinly sliced onion
- 3 cups of chopped green cabbage
- 1 cup of low-sodium vegetable broth
- Freshly ground black pepper, to taste

DIRECTIONS:

1. In a large skillet, heat oil on medium-high heat.
2. Add garlic and then sauté for about 1 minute.
3. Add onion and sauté for about 4-5 minutes.
4. Add cabbage and sauté for about 3-4 minutes.
5. Stir in broth and black pepper and immediately, reduce the heat to low.
6. Cook, covered for about 20 minutes.
7. Serve warm.

Nutrition: *Calories: 45 Fat: 1.8g Carbs: 6.6g Protein: 1.1g Fiber: 1.9g Potassium: 136mg Sodium: 46mg*

SALAD WITH STRAWBERRIES AND GOAT CHEESE

INGREDIENTS:

- Baby lettuce, to taste
- 1-pint strawberries
- Balsamic vinegar
- Extra virgin olive oil
- 1/4 teaspoon black pepper
- 8-ounce soft goat cheese

DIRECTIONS:

1. Prepare the lettuce by washing and drying it, then cut the strawberries.
2. Cut the soft goat cheese into 8 pieces.
3. Put together the balsamic vinegar and the extra virgin olive oil in a large cup with a whisk.
4. Mix the strawberries pressing them and putting them in a bowl, add the dressing and mix, then divide the lettuce into four dishes and cut the other strawberries, arranging them on the salad.
5. Put cheese slices on top and add pepper. Serve and enjoy!

Nutrition: *Calories: 300 Protein: 13g Sodium: 285mg Potassium: 400mg Phosphorus: 193mg*

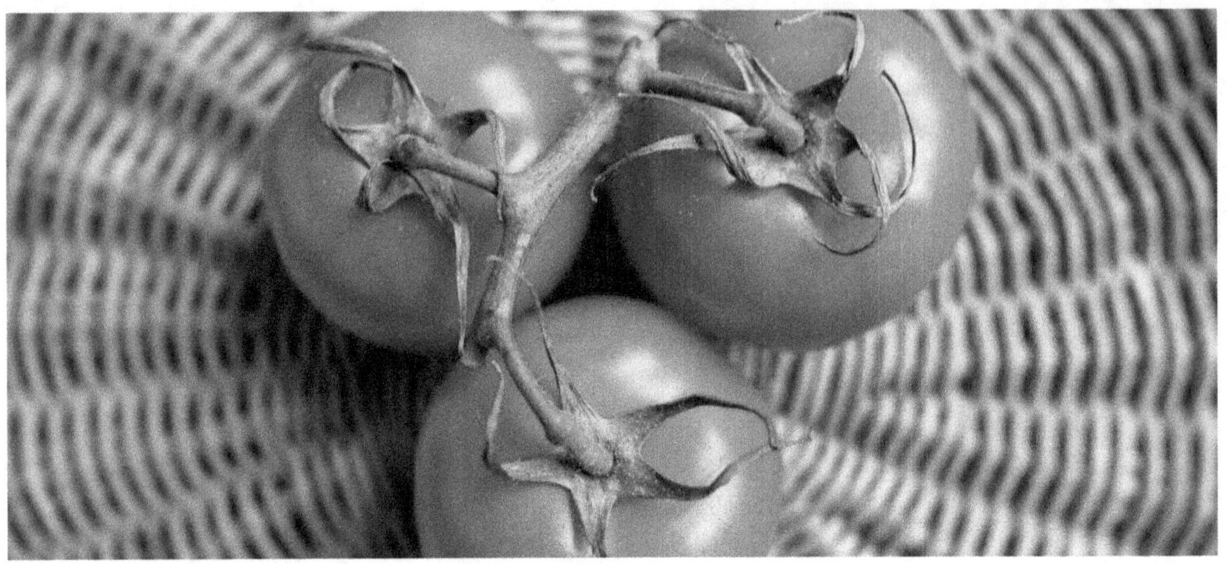

ROASTED VEGGIES MEDITERRANEAN STYLE

INGREDIENTS:

- ½ teaspoon freshly grated lemon zest
- 1 cup grape tomatoes
- 1 tablespoon extra-virgin olive oil
- 1 tablespoon lemon juice
- 1 teaspoon dried oregano
- 10 pitted black olives, sliced
- 12-ounce broccoli crowns, trimmed and cut into bite-sized pieces
- 2 garlic cloves, minced
- 2 teaspoons capers, rinsed

DIRECTIONS:

1. Preheat oven to 350oF and grease a baking sheet with cooking spray.
2. In a large bowl toss together until thoroughly coated salt, garlic, oil, tomatoes and broccoli. Spread broccoli on prepped baking sheet and bake for 8 to 10 minutes.
3. In another large bowl mix capers, oregano, olives, lemon juice, and lemon zest. Mix in roasted vegetables and serve while still warm.

Nutrition: *Calories: 110 Carbs: 16g Protein: 6g Fats: 4g Phosphorus: 138mg Potassium: 745mg Sodium: 214mg*

APPLE SPICE

PORK CHOPS

INGREDIENTS:

DIRECTIONS:

- 1 pound of pork chops
- 2 tablespoons of unsalted butter
- ¼ cup of brown sugar
- ¼ teaspoon of salt (or exclude to reduce sodium)
- ¼ teaspoon of pepper
- ¼ teaspoon of nutmeg
- ¼ teaspoon of cinnamon

2 medium tart of apples

1. Preheat oven to broil.
2. Peel, and slice the apples.
3. Broil the pork chops in the oven for about 4 to 5 minutes on both sides.
4. Use a skillet to melt in the butter, stirring in the brown sugar, salt, nutmeg, cinnamon, pepper, and apples.
5. Cover and cook until the apples become tender and the sauce starts to thicken.
6. Spoon out the sauce over the cooked chops and serve.

Tips:
Marinate the pork chops in the apple juice, pepper, and chopped garlic for additional flavor
Hot skillet can also be used to cook the pork chops instead of broiling. To do this, simply brush the chops with oil and cook for about 5 minutes on each side

Nutrition: *Calories: 306 Protein: 22g Carbohydrates: 21g Fat: 16g Cholesterol: 88mg Sodium: 192mg Potassium: 473mg Phosphorus: 194mg Fiber: 1.2g*

BEEF BURRITOS

INGREDIENTS:

- ¼ cup of onion
- ¼ cup of green pepper
- 1 pound of lean ground beef
- ¼ cup of low-sodium tomato puree
- ¼ teaspoon of black pepper
- ¼ teaspoon of ground cumin
- 6 burrito size flour tortillas

DIRECTIONS:

1. Chop the onion and green pepper.
2. Brown the ground beef in a medium skillet, and drain on paper towels.
3. Spray the skillet with a non-stick cooking spray, then add the onion and green pepper. Cook for about 3 to 5 minutes or until the vegetables become softened.
4. Add the beef, tomato puree, cumin, and black pepper to the onion and pepper mixture. Mix properly and cook over low heat for about 3 to 5 minutes.
5. Divide beef mixture among the tortillas and rolling tortilla over burrito style. Make sure both ends are first folded so that the mixture doesn't fall off.

Nutrition: *Calories: 265 Protein: 15g Carbohydrates: 31g Fat: 9g Cholesterol: 37mg Sodium: 341mg Potassium: 302mg Phosphorus: 171mg Fiber: 1.6g*

CHINESE BEEF WRAPS

INGREDIENTS:

- 2 iceberg lettuce leaves
- ½ diced cucumber
- 1 teaspoon canola oil
- 5-ounce lean ground beef
- 1 teaspoon ground ginger
- 1 tablespoon chili flakes
- 1 minced garlic clove
- 1 tablespoon rice wine vinegar

DIRECTIONS:

1. Mix the ground meat with the garlic, rice wine vinegar, chili flakes and ginger in a bowl.
2. Heat oil in a skillet over medium heat.
3. Add the beef to the pan and cook for 20-25 minutes or until cooked through.
4. Serve beef mixture with diced cucumber in each lettuce wrap and fold.

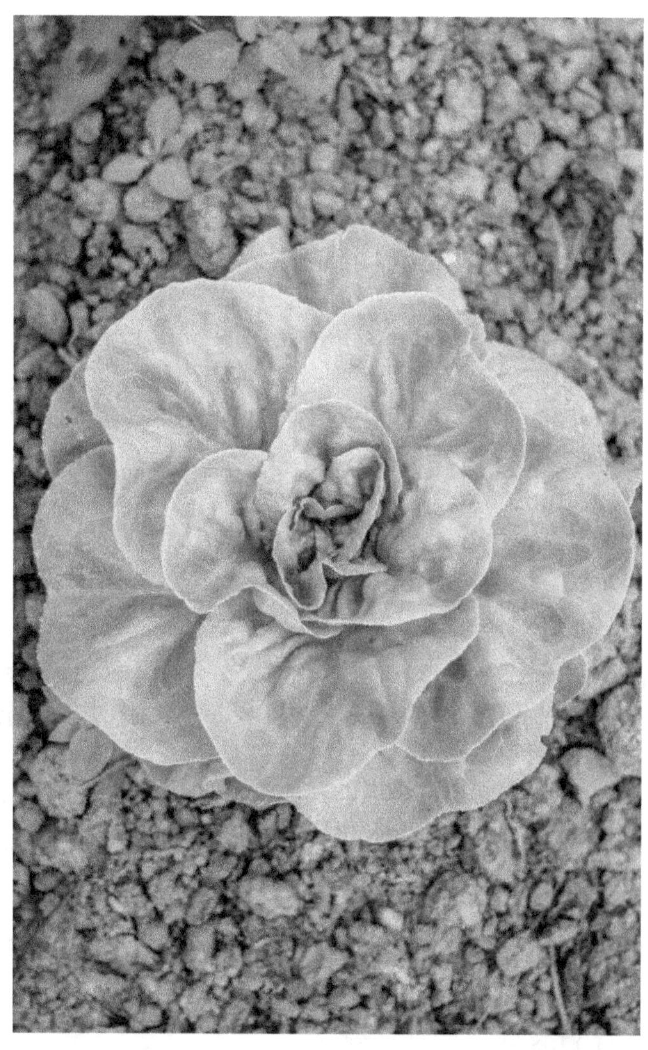

Nutrition: *Calories: 156 Fat: 2g Carbs: 4g Phosphorus: 1mg Sodium (Na): 54mg Protein 14g*

THREE-PEA SALAD WITH GINGER-LIME VINAIGRETTE

INGREDIENTS:

- 1 cup sugar snap peas
- 1 cup snow peas
- 1 cup fresh or thawed frozen sweet peas
- Vinaigrette:
- 1 teaspoon soy sauce, reduced-sodium
- ¼ cup fresh lime juice
- 1 teaspoon fresh lime zest
- 2 teaspoons fresh ginger, chopped
- ½ cup canola oil (can substitute grapeseed oil)
- 1 tablespoon hot sesame oil
- 1 tablespoon sesame seeds
- Optional garnish: freshly cracked coarse black pepper to taste

DIRECTIONS:

1. Lightly toast the sesame seeds in a hot skillet, tossing them constantly for about 3–5 minutes.
2. In a large pot of boiling water over high heat, blanch all 3 types of peas for 2 minutes, drain and then shock them in a bowl of cold water. Transfer to a strainer and drain thoroughly.
3. In a small bowl, whisk the soy sauce, black pepper, lime juice and zest until well-blended, about 1–2 minutes.
4. Continue to whisk, adding the ginger. Slowly drizzle in the canola or grapeseed oil, then add the sesame oil, mixing until well incorporated.
5. In a large bowl, combine the salad dressing with the pea mixture. Toss with the sesame seeds, add the black pepper to taste and serve.

Nutrition: *Calories: 225kcal Total Fat: 21g Saturated Fat: 2g Cholesterol: 0mg Sodium: 70mg Total Carbs: 6g Fiber: 0g Sugar: 0g Protein: 3g*

LEMON ORZO SPRING SALAD

INGREDIENTS:

- ¾ cup or ¼ box orzo pasta
- ¼ cup fresh yellow peppers, diced
- ¼ cup fresh red peppers, diced
- ¼ cup fresh green peppers, diced
- ½ cup fresh red or Vidalia onion, diced
- 2 cups fresh zucchini, medium-cubed
- ¼ cup and 2 tablespoons olive oil
- 3 tablespoons fresh lemon juice
- 1 teaspoon lemon zest
- 3 tablespoons grated Parmesan cheese
- 2 tablespoons fresh rosemary, chopped
- ½ teaspoon black pepper
- ½ teaspoon dried oregano
- ½ teaspoon red pepper flakes

DIRECTIONS:

1. Cook orzo pasta according to box directions, drain, and let sit. (Do not rinse.)
2. Sauté peppers, onions, and zucchini on medium-high heat with 2 tablespoons of oil in a large pan until translucent.
3. Mix lemon juice, lemon zest, ¼ cup olive oil, cheese, rosemary, pepper, oregano and red pepper flakes in a large bowl.
4. Add sautéed vegetables and orzo pasta into the large bowl and fold gently until well mixed.
5. Chill or serve at room temperature.

Nutrition: *Calories: 330kcal Total Fat: 22g Saturated Fat: 4g Cholesterol: 3mg Sodium: 79mg Total Carbs: 28g Fiber: 0g Sugar: 0g Protein: 6g*

HERB-ROASTED
PORK TENDERLOIN

INGREDIENTS:

- 2 garlic cloves
- 1 teaspoon of dried rosemary
- 1 teaspoon of dried thyme
- 1 teaspoon of dried basil
- 1 teaspoon of dried parsley
- 2 teaspoons of black pepper
- 2 tablespoons of Dijon mustard
- 2 (12-ounce) pork tenderloins
- 1½ tablespoons of vegetable oil

DIRECTIONS:

1. Mince the garlic cloves, then add in a small bowl alongside the spices and mustard. Mix thoroughly.
2. Rub the mixture of herb evenly over the pork tenderloins. Cover and refrigerate for about 2 hours.
3. Preheat oven to 400° F.
4. Use a large skillet to heat oil over medium-high heat. Place the tenderloins inside the heated oil and brown all the sides. Remove from skillet and place onto a baking dish without making contact with each other.

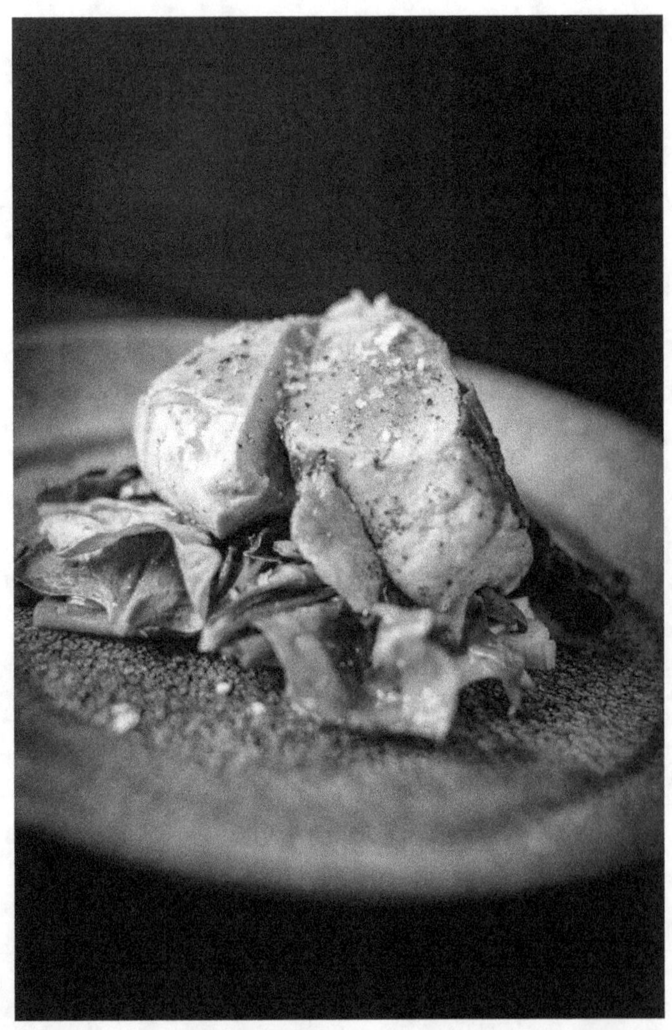

5. Bake tenderloins for about 20 minutes or until 160° F (medium) to 170° F (well done) is registered on the meat thermometer.
6. Set the tenderloins aside to rest for about 10 to 15 minutes before carving. This will help distribute the juices throughout the meat.

Tips: If you are on a low protein diet, reduce the serving size to match your meal plan

Nutrition: *Calories: 178 Protein: 24g Carbohydrates: 1g Fat: 8g Cholesterol: 67mg Sodium: 160mg Potassium: 401mg Phosphorus: 230mg Fiber: 0.4g*

ASIAN ORANGE CHICKEN

INGREDIENTS:

- 1¾ cups of water
- 2 tablespoons of orange juice
- ¼ cup of lemon juice
- ⅓ cup of unseasoned rice vinegar
- 2 tablespoons of reduced-sodium soy sauce
- 1 tablespoon of orange zest
- ⅓ cup packed of brown sugar
- ½ teaspoon of fresh ginger root
- 1 garlic clove
- 2 tablespoons of green onion
- ¼ teaspoon of red pepper flakes
- ½ pound of boneless, and skinless chicken breasts
- 2½ tablespoons of cornstarch
- 3 tablespoons of olive oil

DIRECTIONS:

1. Mince the ginger root and garlic, and chop the green onion.
2. Pour 1½ cups of water, lemon juice, orange juice, rice vinegar, and soy sauce into a saucepan and heat over medium-high heat. Stir in the orange zest, ginger, brown sugar, garlic, chopped onion, and the red pepper flakes, then bring to a boil. Remove from the heat, and allow it to cool for about 10 to 15 minutes.
3. Cut the chicken into ½-inch pieces and place them into a sealable plastic bag. Pour 1 cup of the sauce from step 2 into the bag, reserve the rest of the sauce, seal the bag, and refrigerate for about 2 hours.
4. Use a large skillet to heat olive oil over medium heat, then place the marinated chicken inside the skillet, browning each side. Drain over paper towels and set aside.
5. Clean out the skillet, add in the remaining sauce from step 3, and bring to a boil over medium-high heat. Mix the cornstarch and the remaining cups of water, and stir into the sauce. Reduce the heat to medium-low, and add the pieces of chicken, then simmer for about 5 minutes. Stir occasionally.
6. Cut into four portions and serve hot.

Tips: To complete the meal, serve with steamed rice.
Chicken breast can be substituted for turkey cutlets, pork loin, or chicken thigh meat.
Nutrition: *Calories: 242 Protein: 14g Carbohydrates: 19g Fat: 12g Cholesterol: 37mg Sodium: 340mg Potassium: 240mg Phosphorus: 118mg Fiber: 0.4g*

GARLIC CHICKEN WITH BALSAMIC VINEGAR

INGREDIENTS:

- 4 boneless, and skinless chicken breasts
- 1 teaspoon of fresh ground black pepper
- 1 tablespoon of olive oil
- 8 peeled garlic cloves
- ¾ cup of white button mushrooms, sliced
- ¼ cup of balsamic vinegar
- ¾ cup of low-sodium chicken broth
- 1 bay leaf
- ¼ teaspoon of thyme leaves
- 1 tablespoon of cornstarch

DIRECTIONS:

1. Wash the chicken breasts, trim excess fat, and coat each side with pepper.
2. Use a non-stick skillet and heat the olive oil medium-high heat. Cook for about 3 minutes or until it is browned.
3. Add in the garlic, spread the mushrooms over, and turn the chicken around to prevent it from sticking to the mushroom. Cook for about 3 minutes.
4. Mix the balsamic vinegar, low-sodium chicken broth, thyme leaves, cornstarch and the bay leaf in a small bowl.
5. Add the mixture to the skillet with chicken, and stir until the sauce is thickened.
6. Cover and cook for about 10 minutes over medium-low heat.
7. Remove the bay leaf and garlic, and serve with rice or pasta.

Nutrition: *Calories: 211 Protein: 30g Carbohydrates: 7g Fat: 7g Cholesterol: 73mg Sodium: 88mg Potassium: 337mg Phosphorus: 230mg Fiber: 0.5g*

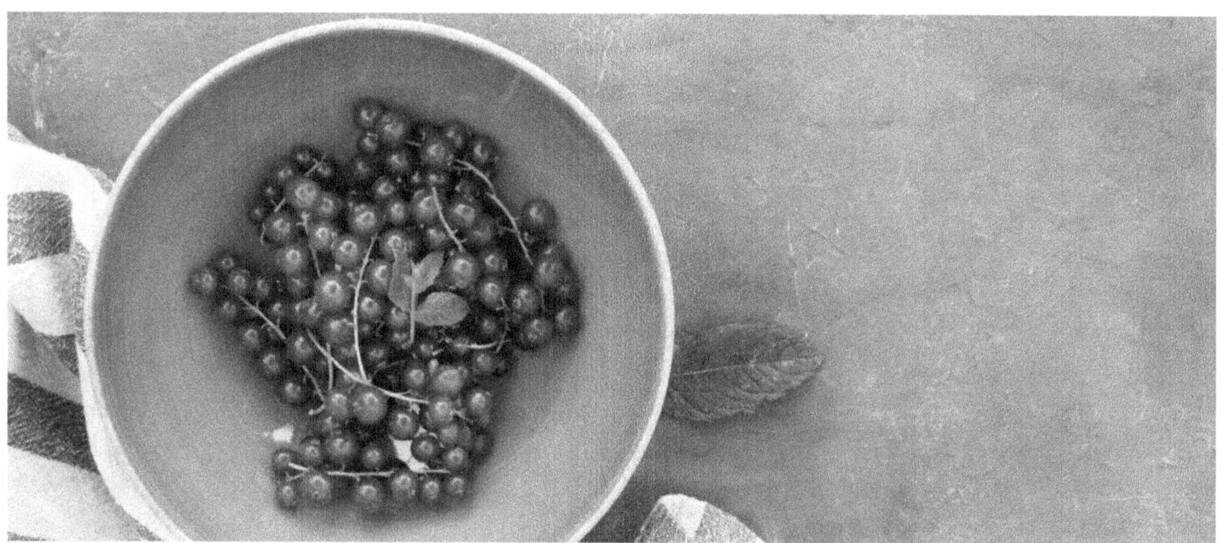

TURKEY BREAST WITH CRANBERRY GRAVY

INGREDIENTS:

- ¼ cup of onion
- ⅓ cup of celery
- 2 cups of carrots
- 18 ounces of boneless, skinless turkey breast
- 1 teaspoon of poultry seasoning
- ½ teaspoon of chicken bouillon granules
- 1 cup of cranberry sauce

DIRECTIONS:

1. Dice the onion, and slice the celery and carrots.
2. Spray a slow cooker with a non-stick cooking spray, place in the turkey breast, sprinkling with poultry seasoning and bouillon granules.
3. Spoon out the cranberry sauce over the top, then add the vegetables from step 1.
4. Cover the slow cooker, and cook for about 4 hours over high heat.
5. Remove and slice the turkey breast, serving with the vegetables and cranberry gravy.

Tips:

You can substitute boneless turkey for a whole turkey breast.

A small portion of regular bouillon gives additional flavor. Controlling the portion helps ensure the sodium content of a low-sodium diet is within the limits.

Nutrition: *Calories: 216 Protein: 18g Carbohydrates: 25g Fat: 6g Cholesterol: 36mg Sodium: 183mg Potassium: 373mg Phosphorus: 187mg Fiber: 2.4g*

GRILLED PINEAPPLE CHICKEN

INGREDIENTS:

- 1 cup of dry sherry
- 1 cup of pineapple juice
- 1 tablespoon of reduced-sodium soy sauce
- 1-¼ pound of skinless, bone-in chicken breast
- 4 pineapple rings

DIRECTIONS:

1. Using a zip-lock bag, place in all the ingredients excluding the pineapple.
2. Refrigerate and marinate overnight.
3. Using an indoor or barbecue grill, place on top of the marinated chicken. Cook for about 15 to 20 minutes or until done, and discard the unused marinade.
4. In the last few minutes of cooking, place the pineapple on top of the grill for about 2 minutes on both sides to heat.
5. Serve each chicken breast, topped with the pineapple.

Tips: Grilling is the recommended method of cooking and is tastier compared to when the chicken is oven-baked.
Cooking sherry and cooking wine both contain high sodium levels; hence, don't substitute the dry sherry in this recipe for either of the two.

Nutrition: *Calories: 211 Protein: 26g Carbohydrates: 20g Fat: 3g Cholesterol: 67mg Sodium: 215mg Potassium: 376mg Phosphorus: 198mg Fiber: 0.5g*

CHICKEN ENCHILADAS

INGREDIENTS:

- 10 ounces of boneless and skinless chicken breasts
- 1 packet of reduced-sodium taco sauce mix
- ⅔ cup of water
- 1 cup of diced red bell pepper
- 6 (6-inch) corn tortillas
- 6 tablespoons of sour cream

DIRECTIONS:

1. Preheat oven to 350° F.
2. Cut the chicken into strips and cook over medium-high heat with a skillet.
3. Mix the taco sauce in a small bowl with ⅔ cup of water.
4. Add in the red bell pepper alongside ⅓ cup of the taco sauce into the skillet. Cook until the chicken is ready.
5. Using a baking dish, spray with a non-stick cooking spray.
6. To prepare the enchiladas, spoon out the chicken and pepper mixture over the tortilla and roll up, then place each of the enchiladas into the baking dish to hold the rolled shape. Pour the remainder of the taco sauce over the top.
7. Bake the enchiladas for about 5 to 7 minutes or until the edges start to brown.
8. Top each of the enchiladas with one tablespoon of sour cream, and serve.

Tips:

Packaged taco seasoning mix has a much lower potassium content than bottled or canned taco seasoning.

Corn tortillas have a moderate phosphorus level. The phosphorous level of enchilada should be kept low by topping with sour cream instead of cheese.

Nutrition: *Calories: 169 Protein: 14g Carbohydrates: 17g Fat: 5g Cholesterol: 37mg Sodium: 367mg Potassium: 215mg Phosphorus: 184mg Fiber: 1.8g*

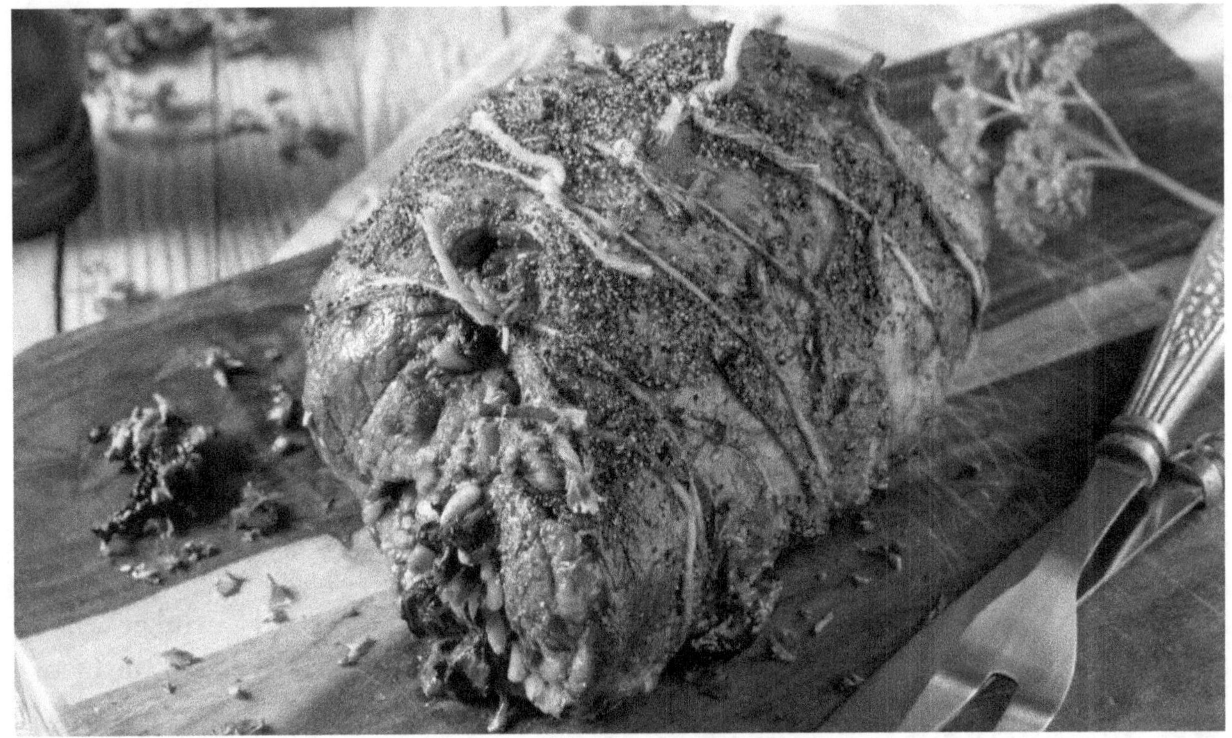

ROASTED LEG OF LAMB

INGREDIENTS:

- 4 tablespoons of unsalted butter
- 1 boneless leg of lamb (4½ pounds) rolled and tied
- ¼ cup of fresh rosemary leaves
- 2 garlic cloves
- 2 tablespoons of dried and crushed oregano leaves
- 1 teaspoon of salt (or exclude to reduce sodium)
- 1 teaspoon of black pepper
- ¼ cup of fresh lemon juice
- 1 cup of water

DIRECTIONS:

1. Preheat oven to 325° F.
2. Set out the butter at room temperature.
3. Wash and slightly trim fat from lamb. Put aside in a roasting pan.
4. Chop the rosemary leaves and mince the garlic.

5. Blend in a bowl the oregano, garlic, rosemary, salt, pepper and half of the soft butter.
6. Cut the leg of lamb into slits, stuffing some of the herb and butter mixture inside the slits, and spreading the remaining herb and butter mixture over the lamb.
7. Mix the lemon juice with the other half butter and pour over the lamb.
8. Cover and bake for about 30 minutes for each pound.
9. After 1 hour, add water to the drippings in the pan. Baste regularly until the meat is tender and browns properly.
10. For crisp skin, uncover the pan during the last half hour.

Tips:
If you are on a low protein diet, reduce the serving size to match your meal plan or check with your dietitian.

Nutrition: *Calories: 318 Protein: 30g Carbohydrates: 0g Fat: 22g Cholesterol: 118mg Sodium: 326mg or 114mg without salt Potassium: 394mg Phosphorus: 228mg Fiber: 0.5g*

CRANBERRY PORK CHOPS

INGREDIENTS:

- 6 (4 ounces) boneless pork loin chops
- ¼ teaspoon of ground black pepper
- 2 teaspoons of cornstarch
- 1 cup of cranapple juice
- 2 teaspoons of honey
- ¾ cup of dried, sweetened cranberries
- 1 tablespoon of fresh minced tarragon
- 1 tablespoon of fresh minced parsley
- 3 cups of brown cooked rice

DIRECTIONS:

1. Sprinkle pepper over the pork chops
2. Use a cooking spray to coat a large non-stick skillet, then cook the chops on each side for about 3 to 4 minutes over medium heat or until it is lightly browned
3. Remove the chops from the skillet and keep warm
4. Mix the cornstarch, juice, and honey in a small bowl until it becomes smooth, then add to the skillet. Stir to loosen browned bits
5. Add and stir in the cranberries, tarragon, and parsley, then bring to a boil. Cook for 2 minutes or until it is thickened and bubbly
6. Add the pork loins to the pan. Cover and reduce the heat, simmering for about 4 to 6 minutes or until the meat thermometer reads 160° F
7. Serve with hot brown rice

Nutrition: *Calories: 397 Protein: 25g Carbohydrates: 45g Fat: 13g Cholesterol: 64mg Sodium: 76mg Potassium: 410mg Phosphorus: 267mg Fiber: 2.7g*

AUTHENTIC

SHRIMP WRAPS

INGREDIENTS:

- 1 tbsp. of olive oil
- 1 minced garlic clove
- 1 seeded and chopped medium red bell pepper
- ½ pound of peeled, deveined and chopped medium shrimp
- Pinch of salt
- Freshly ground black pepper, to taste
- For Wraps:
- 4 large lettuce leaves

DIRECTIONS:

1. In a large skillet, heat oil on medium heat.
2. Add garlic and sauté for about 30 seconds.
3. Add bell pepper and cook for about 2-3 minutes.
4. Add shrimp and seasoning and cook for about 2-3 minutes.
5. Remove from heat and cool slightly. Divide shrimp mixture over lettuce leaves evenly. Serve immediately.

Nutrition: *Calories: 97 Fat: 4.3g Carbs: 3g Protein: 12.6g Fiber: 0.5g Potassium: 81mg Sodium: 169mg*

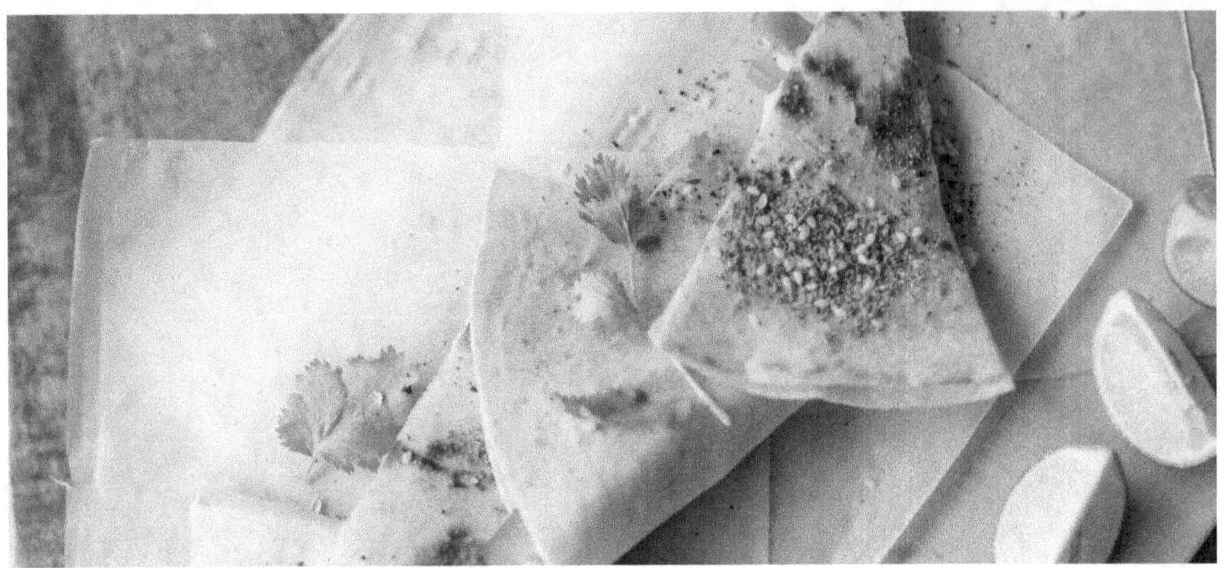

LOVEABLE TORTILLAS

INGREDIENTS:

- ½ cup of low-sodium mayonnaise
- 1 finely minced small garlic clove
- 8-ounce of chopped unsalted cooked chicken
- ½ of seeded and chopped red bell pepper
- ½ of seeded and chopped green bell pepper
- 1 chopped red onion
- 4 (6-ounce) warmed corn tortillas

DIRECTIONS:

1. In a bowl, mix mayonnaise and garlic.
2. In another bowl, mix chicken and vegetables.
3. Arrange the tortillas onto a smooth surface.
4. Spread mayonnaise mixture over each tortilla evenly.
5. Place chicken mixture over ¼ of each tortilla.
6. Fold the outside edges inward and roll up like a burrito.
7. Secure each tortilla with toothpicks to secure the filling.
8. Cut each tortilla in half and serve.

Nutrition: *Calories: 296 Fat: 8.2g Carbs: 44g Protein: 13.5g Fiber: 5.9g Potassium: 262mg Sodium: 162mg*

ELEGANT VEGGIE TORTILLAS

INGREDIENTS:

- 1½ cups of chopped broccoli florets
- 1½ cups of chopped cauliflower florets
- 1 tbsp. of water
- 2 tsp. of canola oil
- 1½ cups of chopped onion
- 1 minced garlic clove
- 2 tbsp. of finely chopped fresh parsley
- 1 cup of low-cholesterol liquid egg substitute
- Freshly ground black pepper, to taste
- 4 (6-ounce) warmed corn tortillas

DIRECTIONS:

1. In a microwave bowl, place broccoli, cauliflower and water and microwave, covered for about 3-5 minutes.
2. Remove from the microwave and drain any liquid.
3. In a skillet, heat oil on medium heat.
4. Add onion and sauté for about 4-5 minutes.
5. Add garlic and sauté for about 1 minute.
6. Stir in broccoli, cauliflower, parsley, egg substitute and black pepper.
7. Reduce the heat to medium-low and simmer for about 10 minutes.
8. Remove from heat and keep aside to cool slightly.
9. Place broccoli mixture over ¼ of each tortilla.
10. Fold the outside edges inward and roll up like a burrito.
11. Secure each tortilla with toothpicks to secure the filling.
12. Cut each tortilla in half and serve.

Nutrition: *Calories: 217 Fat: 3.3g Carbs: 41g Protein: 8.1g Fiber: 6.3g Potassium: 289mg Sodium: 87mg*

DELIGHTFUL PIZZA

INGREDIENTS:

- 2 (6½-inch) pita breads
- 3 tbsp. of low-sodium tomato sauce
- 3-ounce of cubed unsalted cooked chicken
- ¼ cup of chopped onion
- 2 tbsp. of crumbled feta cheese

DIRECTIONS:

1. Preheat the oven to 350 degrees F. Grease a baking sheet.
2. Arrange the pita breads onto a prepared baking sheet.
3. Spread the barbecue sauce over pita bread evenly.
4. Top with chicken and onion evenly and sprinkle with cheese.
5. Bake for about 11-13 minutes.
6. Cut each pizza in half and serve.

Nutrition: *Calories: 133 Fat: 2g Carbs: 18.2g Protein: 9.8g Fiber: 1g Sodium: 287mg*

WINNER KABOBS

INGREDIENTS:

- 1 pound of cubed skinless, boneless chicken breast
- 1 seeded and cut into 1-inch pieces medium red bell pepper
- 1 seeded and cut into 1-inch pieces medium green bell pepper
- 20-ounce of cut into 1-inch pieces pineapple
- 1 cut into 1-inch pieces red onion
- 1/3 cup of low-sodium barbecue sauce
- Freshly ground black pepper, to taste

DIRECTIONS:

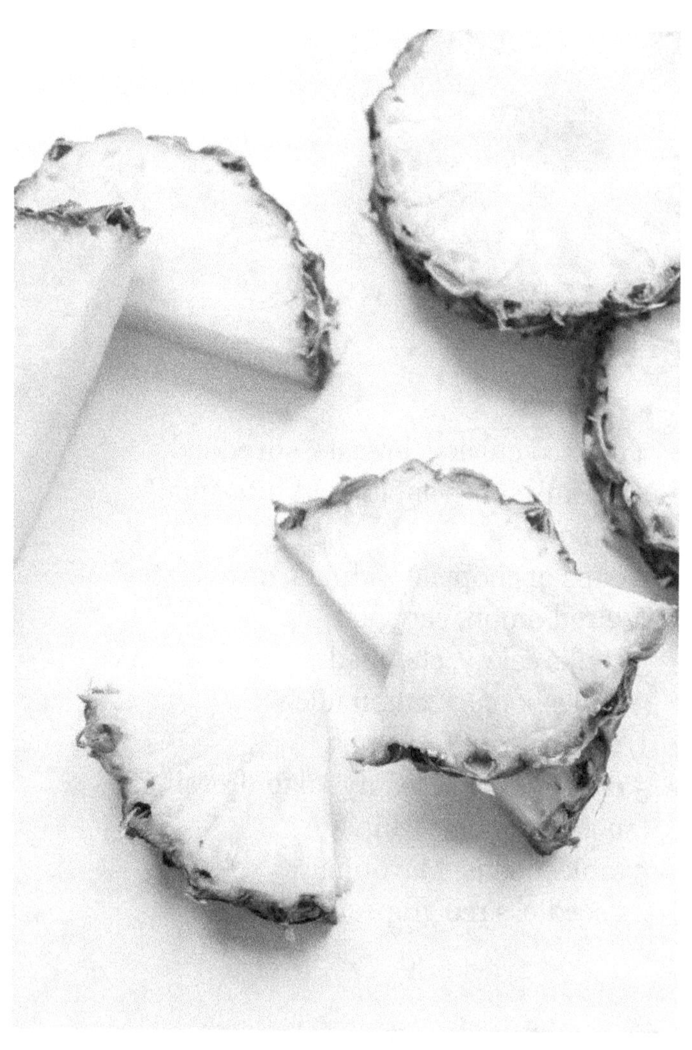

1. Preheat the outdoor grill to medium-high heat. Lightly, grease the grill grate.
2. Thread chicken, bell peppers, pineapple and onion onto pre-soaked 6 wooden skewers.
3. Coat all the ingredients with ½ of barbecue sauce and sprinkle with black pepper.
4. Place the skewers in a prepared baking sheet in a single layer.
5. Grill the skewers for about 9-10 minutes, flipping occasionally.
6. Remove from grill and immediately, coat with remaining barbecue sauce. Serve immediately.

Nutrition:*Calories: 182 Fat: 3g Carbs: 22.2g Protein: 18g Fiber: 2.3g Potassium: 234mg Sodium: 185mg*

PREPARATION: 25 MIN   **COOKING:** 25 MIN   **SERVINGS:** 12

CHICKEN SALAD WITH APPLES, GRAPES, AND WALNUTS

INGREDIENTS:

- 4 cooked chicken breasts, shredded
- 2 granny smith apples, cut into small chunks
- 2 cups of chopped walnuts, or to taste
- 1/2 red onion, chopped
- 3 stalks celery, chopped
- 3 tablespoons. Lemon juice
- 1/2cup of vanilla yogurt
- 5 tablespoons. Creamy salad dressing (such as miracle whip®)
- 5 tablespoons. Mayonnaise
- 25 seedless red grapes, halved

DIRECTIONS:

1. In a big bowl, toss together the shredded chicken, lemon juice, apple chunks, celery, red onion, and walnuts.
2. Get another bowl and whisk together the dressing, vanilla yogurt, and mayonnaise. Pour over the chicken mixture. Toss to coat. Fold the grapes carefully into the salad.

Nutrition: *Calories: 307 Total fat: 22.7g Carbohydrates: 10.8g Protein: 17.3g Cholesterol: 41mg Sodium: 128mg*

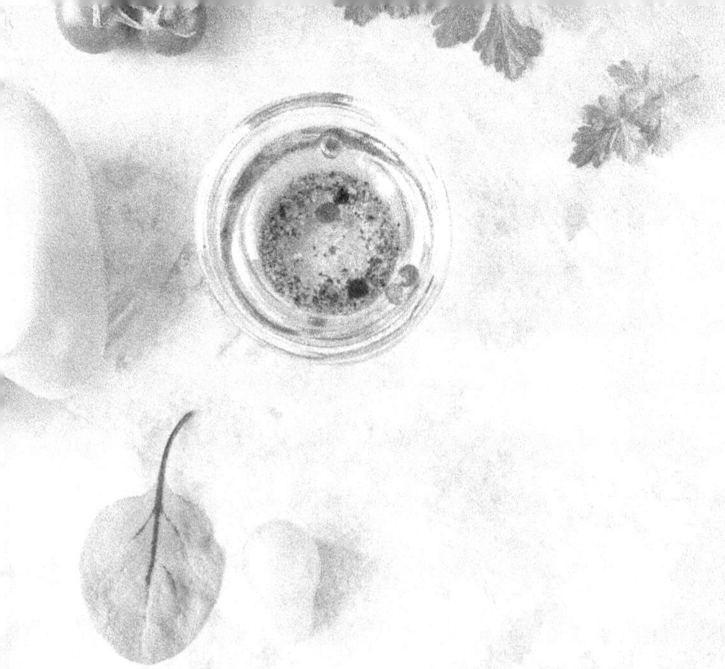

CHAPTER 7

<u>Dinner Recipes</u>

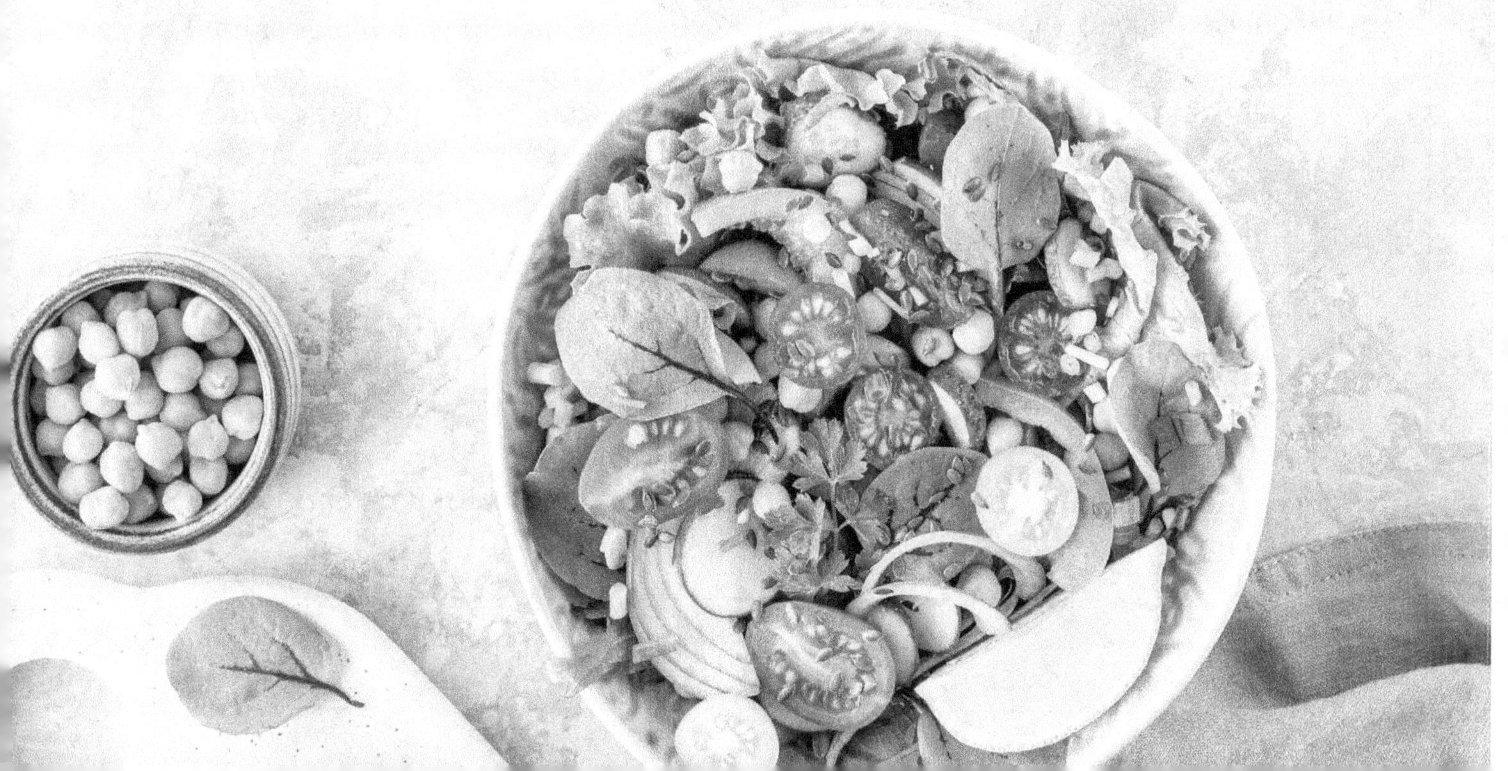

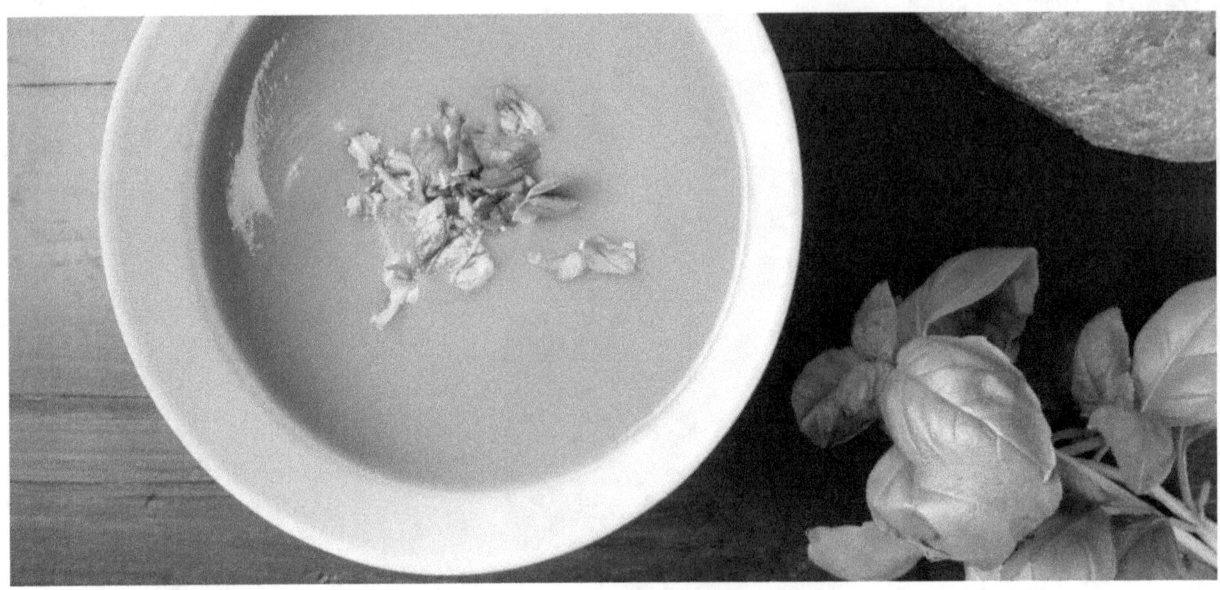

EGGPLANT AND

RED PEPPER SOUP

INGREDIENTS:

- Sweet onion – 1 small, cut into quarters
- Small red bell peppers – 2, halved
- Cubed eggplant – 2 cups
- Garlic – 2 cloves, crushed
- Olive oil – 1 Tbsp.
- Chicken stock – 1 cup
- Water
- Chopped fresh basil – ¼ cup
- Ground black pepper

DIRECTIONS:

1. Preheat the oven to 350°F.
2. Put the onions, red peppers, eggplant, and garlic in a baking dish.
3. Drizzle the vegetables with the olive oil.
4. Roast the vegetables for 30 minutes or until they are slightly charred and soft.
5. Cool the vegetables slightly and remove the skin from the peppers.
6. Puree the vegetables with a hand mixer (with the chicken stock).
7. Transfer the soup to a medium pot and add enough water to reach the desired thickness.
8. Heat the soup to a simmer and add the basil.
9. Season with pepper and serve.

Nutrition: *Calories: 61 Fat: 2g Carb: 9g Phosphorus: 33mg Potassium: 198mg Sodium: 98mg Protein: 2g*

SEAFOOD CASSEROLE

INGREDIENTS:

- Eggplant – 2 cups, peeled and diced into 1-inch pieces
- Butter, for greasing the baking dish
- Olive oil – 1 tbsp.
- Sweet onion – ½, chopped
- Minced garlic – 1 tsp.
- Celery stalk – 1, chopped
- Red bell pepper – ½, boiled and chopped
- Freshly squeezed lemon juice – 3 Tbsps.
- Hot sauce – 1 tsp.
- Creole seasoning mix – ¼ tsp.
- White rice – ½ cup, uncooked
- Egg – 1 large
- Cooked shrimp – 4 ounces
- Queen crab meat – 6 ounces

DIRECTIONS:

1. Preheat the oven to 350°F.
2. Boil the eggplant in a saucepan for 5 minutes. Drain and set aside.
3. Grease a 9-by-13-inch baking dish with butter and set aside.
4. Heat the olive oil in a large skillet over medium heat.
5. Sauté the garlic, onion, celery, and bell pepper for 4 minutes or until tender.
6. Add the sautéed vegetables to the eggplant, along with the lemon juice, hot sauce, seasoning, rice, and egg.
7. Stir to combine.
8. Fold in the shrimp and crab meat.
9. Spoon the casserole mixture into the casserole dish, patting down the top.
10. Bake for 25 to 30 minutes or until casserole is heated through and rice is tender.
11. Serve warm.

Nutrition: *Calories: 118 Fat: 4g Carb: 9g Phosphorus: 102mg Potassium: 199mg Sodium: 235mg Protein: 12g*

GROUND BEEF
AND RICE SOUP

INGREDIENTS:

- Extra-lean ground beef – ½ pound
- Small sweet onion – ½, chopped
- Minced garlic – 1 tsp.
- Water – 2 cups
- Low-sodium beef broth – 1 cup
- Long-grain white rice – ½ cup, uncooked
- Celery stalk – 1, chopped
- Fresh green beans – ½ cup, cut into – 1-inch pieces
- Chopped fresh thyme – 1 tsp.
- Ground black pepper

DIRECTIONS:

1. Sauté the ground beef in a saucepan for 6 minutes or until the beef is completely browned.
2. Drain off the excess fat and add the onion and garlic to the saucepan.
3. Sauté the vegetables for about 3 minutes, or until they are softened.
4. Add the celery, rice, beef broth, and water.
5. Bring the soup to a boil, reduce the heat to low and simmer for 30 minutes or until the rice is tender.
6. Add the green beans and thyme and simmer for 3 minutes.
7. Remove the soup from the heat and season with pepper.

Nutrition: *Calories: 154 Fat: 7g Carb: 14g Phosphorus: 76mg Potassium: 179mg Sodium: 133mg Protein: 9g*

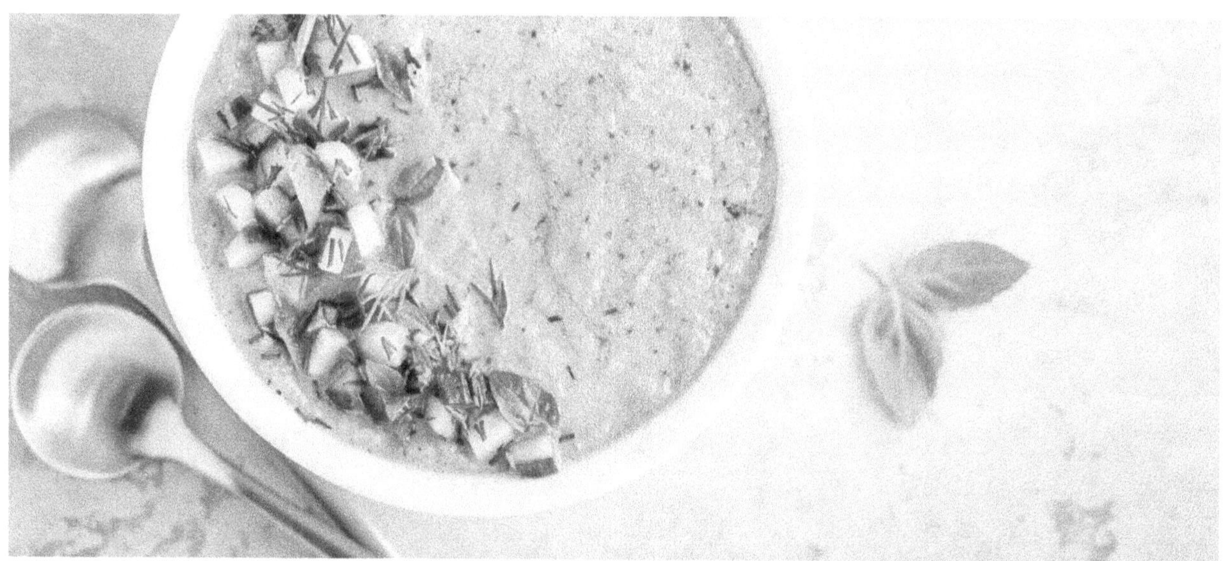

CUCUMBER SOUP

INGREDIENTS:

- 2 medium cucumbers, peeled and diced
- 1/3 cup sweet white onion, diced
- 1 green onion, diced
- 1/4 cup fresh mint
- 2 tablespoon fresh dill
- 2 tablespoon lemon juice
- 2/3 cup water
- 1/2 cup half and half cream
- 1/3 cup sour cream
- 1/2 teaspoon pepper
- Fresh dill sprigs for garnish

DIRECTIONS:

1. Gather all of the ingredients into a food processor and toss.
2. Puree the mixture and refrigerate for 2 hours.
3. Garnish with dill sprigs.
4. Enjoy fresh.

Nutrition: *Calories: 77 Protein: 2g Carbohydrates: 6g Fat: 5g Cholesterol: 12mg Sodium: 128mg Potassium: 258mg Phosphorus: 64mg Calcium: 60mg Fiber: 1.0g*

BAKED FLOUNDER

INGREDIENTS:

- Homemade mayonnaise – ¼ cup
- Juice of 1 lime
- Zest of 1 lime
- Chopped fresh cilantro – ½ cup
- Flounder fillets – 4 (3-ounce)
- Ground black pepper

DIRECTIONS:

1. Preheat the oven to 400°F.
2. In a bowl, stir together the cilantro, lime juice, lime zest, and mayonnaise.
3. Place 4 pieces of foil, about 8 by 8 inches square, on a clean work surface.
4. Place a flounder fillet in the center of each square.
5. Top the fillets evenly with the mayonnaise mixture.
6. Season the flounder with pepper.
7. Fold the sides of the foil over the fish, creating a snug packet, and place the foil packets on a baking sheet.
8. Bake the fish for 4 to 5 minutes.
9. Unfold the packets and serve.

Nutrition: *Calories: 92 Fat: 4g Carb: 2g Phosphorus: 208mg Potassium: 137mg Sodium: 267mg Protein: 12g*

PERSIAN CHICKEN

INGREDIENTS:

- Sweet onion – ½, chopped
- Lemon juice – ¼ cup
- Dried oregano – 1 Tbsp.
- Minced garlic – 1 tsp.
- Sweet paprika – 1 tsp.
- Ground cumin – ½ tsp.
- Olive oil – ½ cup
- Boneless, skinless chicken thighs – 5

DIRECTIONS:

1. Put the cumin, paprika, garlic, oregano, lemon juice, and onion in a food processor and pulse to mix the ingredients.
2. Keep the motor running and add the olive oil until the mixture is smooth.
3. Place the chicken thighs in a large sealable freezer bag and pour the marinade into the bag.
4. Seal the bag and place it in the refrigerator, turning the bag twice, for 2 hours.
5. Remove the thighs from the marinade and discard the extra marinade.
6. Preheat the barbecue to medium.
7. Grill the chicken for about 20 minutes, turning once, until it reaches 165F.

Nutrition: *Calories: 321 Fat: 21g Carb: 3g Phosphorus: 131mg Potassium: 220mg Sodium: 86mg Protein: 22g*

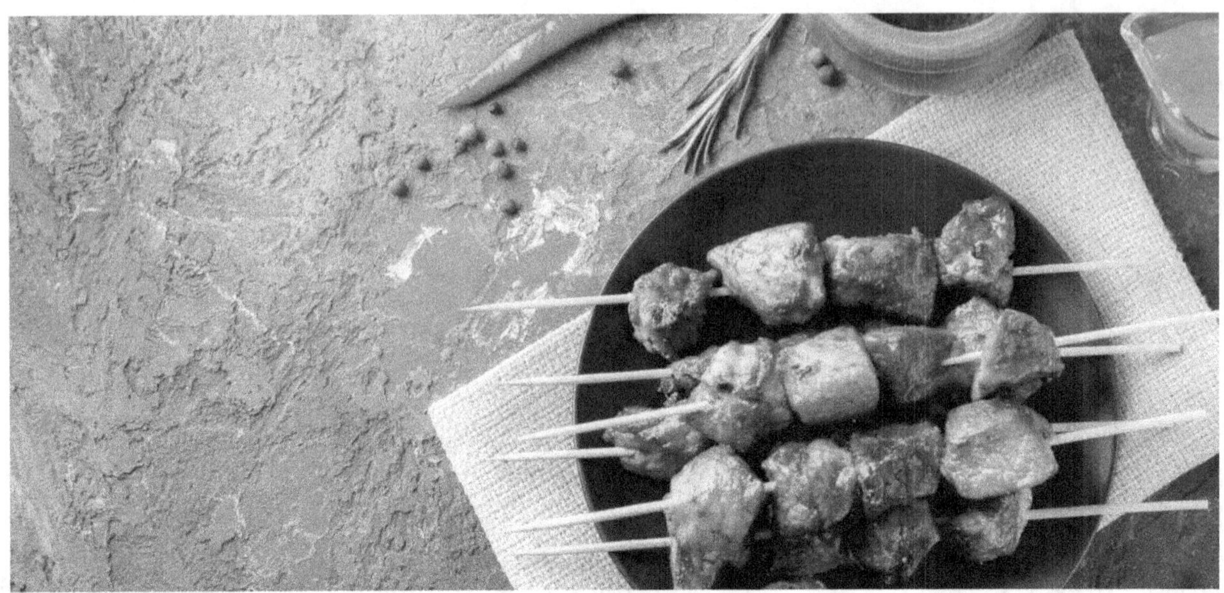

PORK SOUVLAKI

INGREDIENTS:

- Olive oil – 3 Tbsps.
- Lemon juice – 2 Tbsps.
- Minced garlic – 1 tsp.
- Chopped fresh oregano – 1 Tbsp.
- Ground black pepper – ¼ tsp.
- Pork leg – 1 pound, cut in 2-inch cubes

DIRECTIONS:

1. In a bowl, stir together the lemon juice, olive oil, garlic, oregano, and pepper.
2. Add the pork cubes and toss to coat.
3. Place the bowl in the refrigerator, covered, for 2 hours to marinate.
4. Thread the pork chunks onto 8 wooden skewers that have been soaked in water.
5. Preheat the barbecue to medium-high heat.
6. Grill the pork skewers for about 12 minutes, turning once, until just cooked through but still juicy.

Nutrition: *Calories: 95 Fat: 4g Carb: 0g Phosphorus: 125mg Potassium: 230mg Sodium: 29mg Protein: 13g*

SALMON & PESTO SALAD

INGREDIENTS:

For the pesto:

- 1 minced garlic clove
- ½ cup fresh arugula
- ¼ cup extra virgin olive oil
- ½ cup fresh basil
- 1 tsp. black pepper

For the salmon:

- 4 oz. skinless salmon fillet
- 1 tbsp. coconut oil

For the salad:

- ½ juiced lemon
- 2 sliced radishes
- ½ cup iceberg lettuce
- 1 tsp. black pepper

DIRECTIONS:

1. Prepare the pesto by blending all the ingredients for the pesto in a food processor or by grinding with a pestle and mortar. Set aside.
2. Add a skillet to the stove on medium-high heat and melt the coconut oil.
3. Add the salmon to the pan.
4. Cook for 7-8 minutes and turn over.
5. Cook for a further 3-4 minutes or until cooked through.
6. Remove fillets from the skillet and allow to rest.
7. Mix the lettuce and the radishes and squeeze over the juice of ½ lemon.
8. Flake the salmon with a fork and mix through the salad.
9. Toss to coat and sprinkle with a little black pepper to serve.

Nutrition: *Calories: 221 Protein: 13g Carbs: 1g Fat: 34g Sodium: 80mg Potassium: 119 mg, Phosphorus: 158 mg*

CHICKEN STEW

INGREDIENTS:

- Olive oil – 1 Tbsp.
- Boneless, skinless chicken thighs – 1 pound, cut into 1-inch cubes
- Sweet onion – ½, chopped
- Minced garlic – 1 Tbsp.
- Chicken stock – 2 cups
- Water – 1 cup, plus 2 Tbsps.
- Carrot – 1, sliced
- Celery – 2 stalks, sliced
- Turnip – 1, sliced thin
- Chopped fresh thyme – 1 Tbsp.
- Chopped fresh rosemary – 1 tsp.
- Cornstarch – 2 tsps.
- Ground black pepper to taste

DIRECTIONS:

1. Place a large saucepan on medium heat and add the olive oil.
2. Sauté the chicken for 6 minutes or until it is lightly browned, stirring often.
3. Add the onion and garlic, and sauté for 3 minutes.
4. Add 1-cup water, chicken stock, carrot, celery, and turnip and bring the stew to a boil.
5. Reduce the heat to low and simmer for 30 minutes or until the chicken is cooked through and tender.
6. Add the thyme and rosemary and simmer for 3 minutes more.
7. In a small bowl, stir together the 2 tbsps. Of water and the cornstarch; add the mixture to the stew.
8. Stir to incorporate the cornstarch mixture and cook for 3 to 4 minutes or until the stew thickens.
9. Remove from the heat and season with pepper.

Nutrition: *Calories: 141 Fat: 8g Carb: 5g Phosphorus: 53mg Potassium: 192mg Sodium: 214mg Protein: 9g*

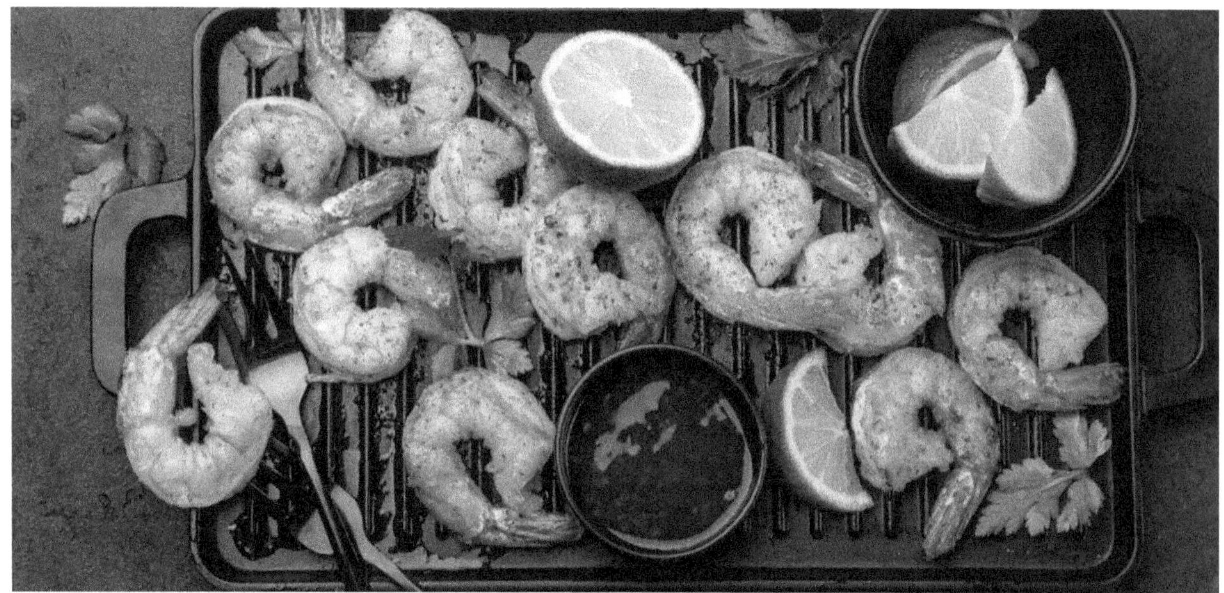

GRILLED SHRIMP WITH CUCUMBER LIME SALSA

INGREDIENTS:

- Olive oil – 2 tbsp.
- Large shrimp – 6 ounces, peeled and deveined, tails left on
- Minced garlic – 1 tsp
- Chopped English cucumber – ½ cup
- Chopped mango – ½ cup
- Zest of 1 lime
- Juice of 1 lime
- Ground black pepper
- Lime wedges for garnish

DIRECTIONS:

1. Soak 4 wooden skewers in water for 30 minutes.
2. Preheat the barbecue to medium heat.
3. In a bowl, toss together the olive oil, shrimp, and garlic.
4. Thread the shrimp onto the skewers, about 4 shrimp per skewer.
5. In a bowl, stir together the mango, cucumber, lime zest, and lime juice, and season the salsa lightly with pepper. Set aside.
6. Grill the shrimp for 10 minutes, turning once or until the shrimp is opaque and cooked through.
7. Season the shrimp lightly with pepper.
8. Serve the shrimp on the cucumber salsa with lime wedges on the side.

Nutrition: *Calories: 120kcal Total Fat: 8g Saturated Fat: 0g Cholesterol: 0mg Sodium: 60mg Total Carbs: 4g Fiber: 0g Sugar: 0g Protein: 9g*

SHRIMP SCAMPI LINGUINE

INGREDIENTS:

- Uncooked linguine – 4 ounces
- Olive oil – 1 tsp.
- Minced garlic – 2 tsp
- Shrimp – 4 ounces, peeled, deveined, and chopped
- Dry white wine – ½ cup
- Juice of 1 lemon
- Chopped fresh basil – 1 tbsp
- Heavy whipping cream – ½ cup
- Ground black pepper

DIRECTIONS:

1. Cook the linguine according to package instructions, drain and set aside.
2. Heat the olive oil in a skillet.
3. Sauté the garlic and shrimp for 6 minutes or until the shrimp is opaque and just cooked through.
4. Add the lemon juice, wine, and basil. Cook for 5 minutes.
5. Stir in the cream and simmer for 2 minutes more.
6. Add the linguine to the skillet and toss to coat.
7. Divide the pasta onto 4 plates to serve.

Nutrition: *Calories: 219kcal Total Fat: 7g Saturated Fat: 0g Cholesterol: 0mg Sodium: 42mg Total Carbs: 21g Fiber: 0g Sugar: 0g Protein: 12g*

CRAB CAKES WITH

LIME SALSA

INGREDIENTS:

- English cucumber – ½, diced
- Lime – 1, chopped
- Boiled and chopped red bell pepper – ½ cup
- Chopped fresh cilantro – 1 tsp
- Ground black pepper
- For the crab cakes
- Queen crab meat – 8 ounces
- Bread crumbs – ¼ cup
- Small egg – 1
- Boiled and chopped red bell pepper – ¼ cup
- Scallion – 1, both green and white parts, minced
- Chopped fresh parsley – 1 tbsp
- Splash hot sauce
- Olive oil spray, for the pan

DIRECTIONS:

1. To make the salsa, in a small bowl stir together the lime, cucumber, red pepper and cilantro. Season with pepper and set aside.
2. To make the crab cakes, in a bowl mix the bread crumbs, crab, red pepper, egg, scallion, parsley, and hot sauce until it holds together. Add more bread crumbs, if necessary.
3. Form the crab mixture into 4 patties and place them on a plate.
4. Refrigerate the crab cakes for 1 hour to firm them.
5. Spray a skillet with olive oil spray and place on medium heat.
6. Cook the crab cakes in batches, turning, for about 5 minutes per side or until golden brown.
7. Serve the crab cakes with salsa.

Nutrition: *Calories: 115kcal Total Fat: 2g Saturated Fat: 0g Cholesterol: 0mg Sodium: 421mg Total Carbs: 7g Fiber: 0g Sugar: 0g Protein: 16g*

SHRIMP WITH SALSA

INGREDIENTS:

- Olive oil – 2 Tbsp.
- Large shrimp – 6 ounces, peeled and deveined, tails left on
- Minced garlic – 1 tsp.
- Chopped English cucumber – ½ cup
- Chopped mango – ½ cup
- Zest of 1 lime
- Juice of 1 lime
- Ground black pepper
- Lime wedges for garnish

DIRECTIONS:

1. Soak 4 wooden skewers in water for 30 minutes.
2. Preheat the barbecue to medium heat.
3. In a bowl, toss together the olive oil, shrimp, and garlic.
4. Thread the shrimp onto the skewers, about 4 shrimp per skewer.
5. In a bowl, stir together the mango, cucumber, lime zest, and lime juice, and season the salsa lightly with pepper. Set aside.
6. Grill the shrimp for 10 minutes, turning once or until the shrimp is opaque and cooked through.
7. Season the shrimp lightly with pepper.
8. Serve the shrimp on the cucumber salsa with lime wedges on the side.

Nutrition: *Calories: 120 Fat: 8g Carb: 4g Phosphorus: 91mg Potassium: 129mg Sodium: 60mg Protein: 9g*

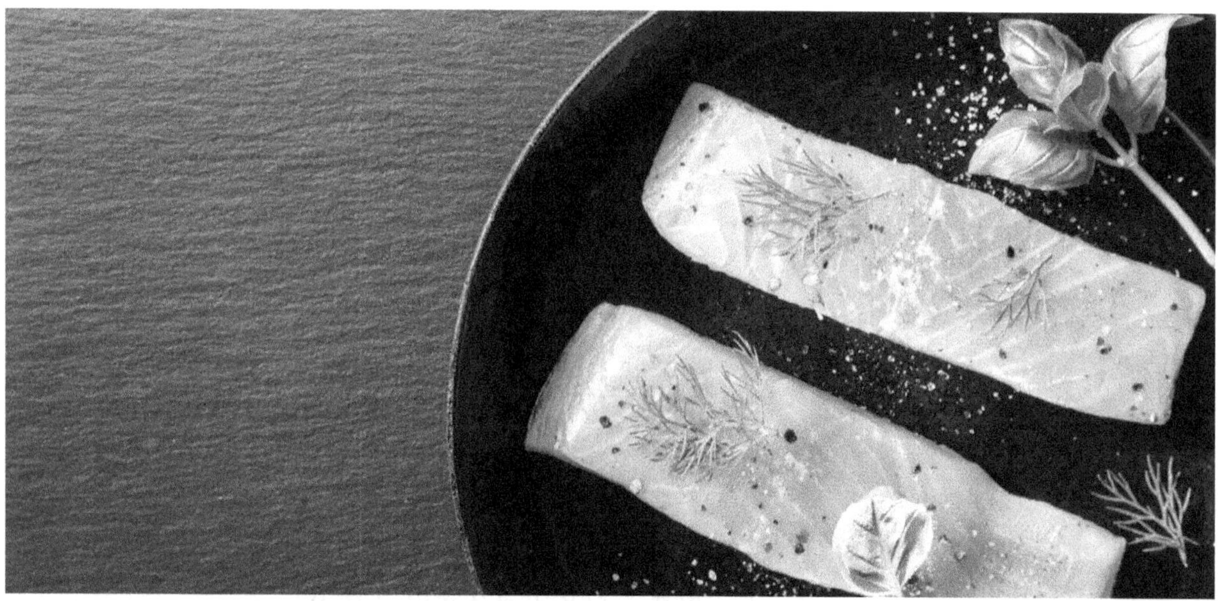

SWEET GLAZED SALMON

INGREDIENTS:

- Honey – 2 tbsp
- Lemon zest – 1 tsp
- Ground black pepper – ½ tsp
- Salmon fillets – 4 (3-ounce) each
- Olive oil – 1 tbsp
- Scallion – ½, white and green parts, chopped

DIRECTIONS:

1. In a bowl, stir together the lemon zest, honey, and pepper.
2. Wash the salmon and pat dry with paper towels.
3. Rub the honey mixture all over each fillet.
4. In a large skillet, heat the olive oil.
5. Add the salmon fillets and cook the salmon for 10 minutes, turning once, or until it is lightly browned and just cooked through.
6. Serve topped with chopped scallion.

Nutrition: *Calories: 240kcal Total Fat: 15g Saturated Fat: 0g Cholesterol: 0mg Sodium: 51mg Total Carbs: 9g Fiber: 0g Sugar: 0g Protein: 17g*

BEEF CHILI

INGREDIENTS:

- Onion – 1, diced
- Red bell pepper – 1, diced
- Garlic – 2 cloves, minced
- Lean ground beef – 6 oz.
- Chili powder – 1 tsp.
- Oregano – 1 tsp.
- Extra virgin olive oil – 2 Tbsps.
- Water – 1 cup
- Brown rice – 1 cup
- Fresh cilantro – 1 Tbsp. to serve

DIRECTIONS:

1. Soak vegetables in warm water.
2. Bring a pan of water to a boil and add rice for 20 minutes.
3. Meanwhile, add the oil to a pan and heat on medium-high heat.
4. Add the pepper, onions, and garlic and sauté for 5 minutes until soft.
5. Remove and set aside.
6. Add the beef to the pan and stir until browned.
7. Add the vegetables back into the pan and stir.
8. Now add the chili powder and herbs and the water, cover and turn the heat down a little to simmer for 15 minutes.
9. Meanwhile, drain the water from the rice, and the lid and steam while the chili is cooking.
10. Serve hot with the fresh cilantro sprinkled over the top.

Nutrition: *Calories: 459 Fat: 22g Carb: 36g Phosphorus: 332mg Potassium: 360mg Sodium: 33mg Protein: 22g*

SHRIMP PAELLA

INGREDIENTS:

- 1 cup cooked brown rice
- 1 chopped red onion
- 1 tsp. paprika
- 1 chopped garlic clove
- 1 tbsp. olive oil
- 6 oz. frozen cooked shrimp
- 1 deseeded and sliced chili pepper
- 1 tbsp. oregano

DIRECTIONS:

1. Heat the olive oil in a large pan on medium-high heat.
2. Add the onion and garlic and sauté for 2-3 minutes until soft.
3. Now add the shrimp and sauté for a further 5 minutes or until hot through.
4. Now add the herbs, spices, chili and rice with 1/2 cup boiling water.
5. Stir until everything is warm and the water has been absorbed.
6. Plate up and serve.

Nutrition: *Calories 221 Protein: 17g Carbs: 31g Fat: 8g Sodium: 235mg Potassium: 176mg Phosphorus: 189mg*

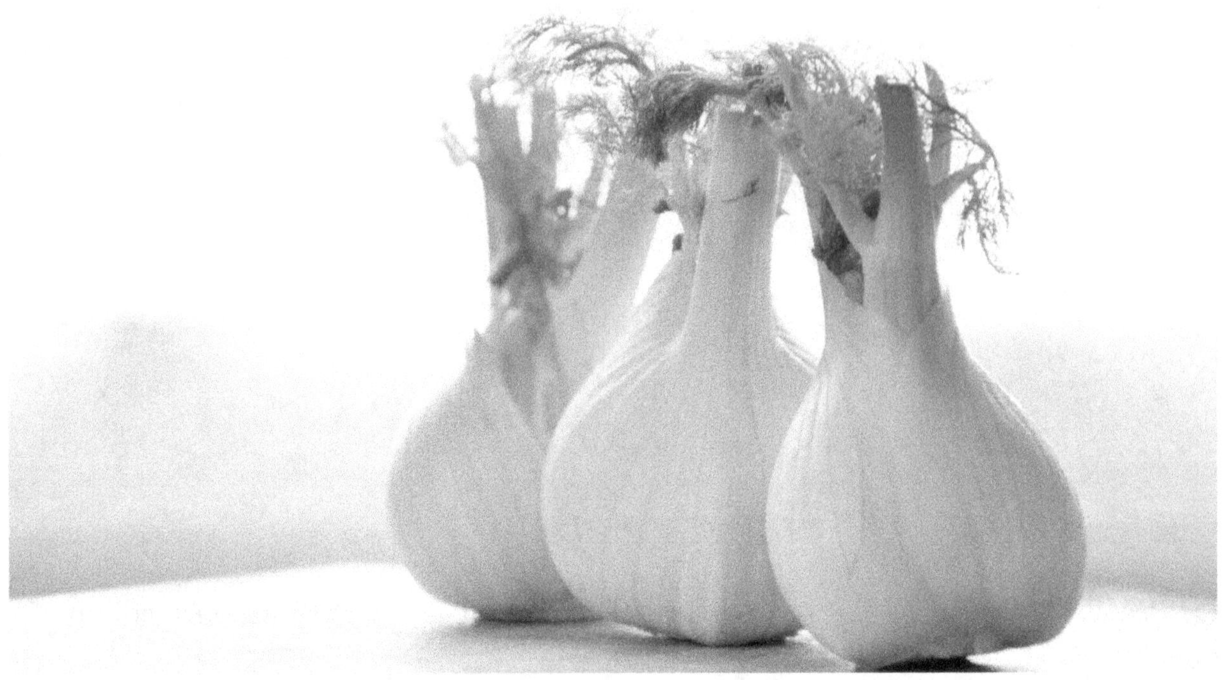

BAKED FENNEL & GARLIC SEA BASS

INGREDIENTS:

- 1 lemon
- ½ sliced fennel bulb
- 6 oz. sea bass fillets
- 1 tsp. black pepper
- 2 garlic cloves

DIRECTIONS:

1. Preheat the oven to 375°F/Gas Mark 5.
2. Sprinkle black pepper over the Sea Bass.
3. Slice the fennel bulb and garlic cloves.
4. Add 1 salmon fillet and half the fennel and garlic to one sheet of baking paper or tin foil.
5. Squeeze in 1/2 lemon juices.
6. Repeat for the other fillet.
7. Fold and add to the oven for 12-15 minutes or until fish is thoroughly cooked through.
8. Meanwhile, add boiling water to your couscous, cover and allow to steam.
9. Serve with your choice of rice or salad.

Nutrition: *Calories : 221Protein: 14g Carbs: 3gFat: 2g Sodium: 119mg Potassium: 398mg Phosphorus: 149mg*

LEMON, GARLIC & CILANTRO TUNA AND RICE

INGREDIENTS:

- ½ cup arugula
- 1 tbsp. extra virgin olive oil
- 1 cup cooked rice
- 1 tsp. black pepper
- ¼ finely diced red onion
- 1 juiced lemon
- 3 oz. canned tuna
- 2 tbsps. Chopped fresh cilantro

DIRECTIONS:

1. Mix the olive oil, pepper, cilantro and red onion in a bowl.
2. Stir in the tuna, cover and leave in the fridge for as long as possible (if you can) or serve immediately.
3. When ready to eat, serve up with the cooked rice and arugula!

Nutrition: *Calories: 221 Protein: 11g Carbs: 26g Fat: 7g Sodium: 143mg Potassium: 197mg Phosphorus: 182mg*

COD & GREEN

BEAN RISOTTO

INGREDIENTS:

- ½ cup arugula
- 1 finely diced white onion
- 4 oz. c od fillet
- 1 cup white rice
- 2 lemon wedges
- 1 cup boiling water
- ¼ tsp. black pepper
- 1 cup low sodium chicken broth
- 1 tbsp. extra virgin olive oil
- ½ cup green beans

DIRECTION:

1. Heat the oil in a large pan on medium heat.
2. Sauté the chopped onion for 5 minutes until soft before adding in the rice and stirring for 1-2 minutes.
3. Combine the broth with boiling water.
4. Add half of the liquid to the pan and stir slowly.
5. Slowly add the rest of the liquid whilst continuously stirring for up to 20-30 minutes.
6. Stir in the green beans to the risotto.
7. Place the fish on top of the rice, cover and steam for 10 minutes.
8. Ensure the water does not dry out and keep topping up until the rice is cooked thoroughly.
9. Use your fork to break up the fish fillets and stir into the rice.
10. Sprinkle with freshly ground pepper to serve and a squeeze of fresh lemon.
11. Garnish with the lemon wedges and serve with the arugula.

Nutrition: *Calories: 221 Protein: 12g Carbs: 29g Fat: 8g Sodium: 398mg Potassium: 347mg Phosphorus: 241mg*

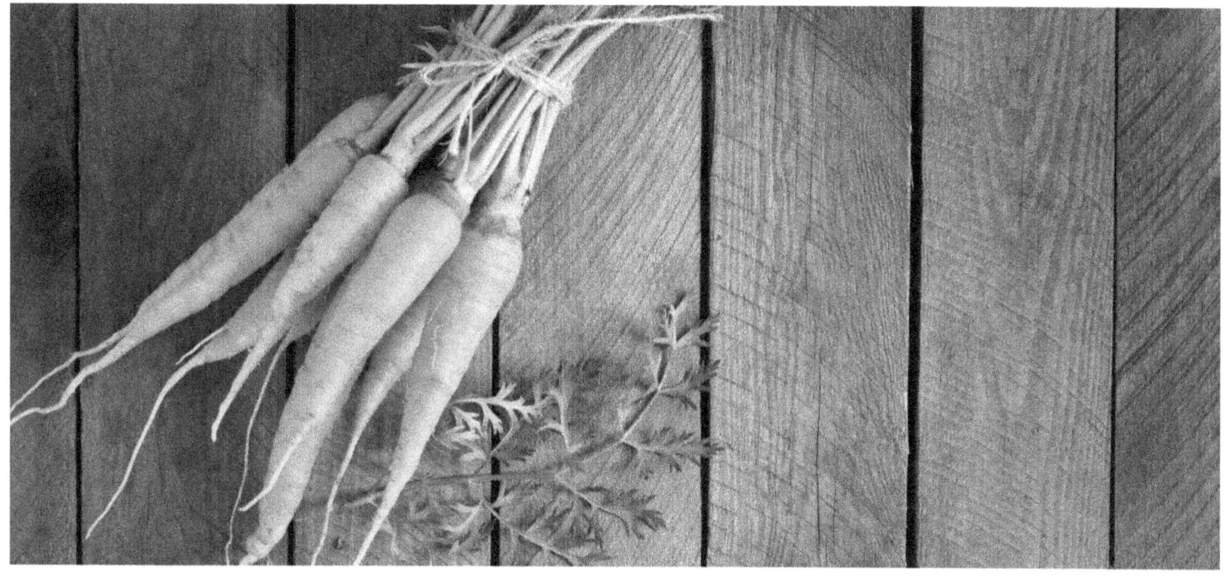

LETTUCE AND CARROT SALAD WITH BALSAMIC VINAIGRETTE

INGREDIENTS:

For the vinaigrette:

- Olive oil – ½ cup
- Balsamic vinegar – 4 tbsp
- Chopped fresh oregano – 2 tbsp
- Pinch red pepper flakes
- Ground black pepper

For the salad:

- Shredded green leaf lettuce – 4 cups
- Carrot – 1, shredded
- Fresh green beans – ¾ cup, cut into 1-inch pieces
- Large radishes – 3, sliced thinly

DIRECTIONS:

1. To make the vinaigrette: place the vinaigrette ingredients in a bowl and whisk.
2. To make the salad: in a bowl, toss together the carrot, lettuce, green beans, and radishes.
3. Add the vinaigrette to the vegetables and toss to coat.
4. Arrange the salad on plates and serve.

Nutrition: *Calories: 273   Fat: 27g   Carb: 7g Phosphorus: 30mg Potassium: 197mg Sodium: 27mg Protein: 1g*

CUCUMBERS WITH SOUR CREAM

INGREDIENTS:

- 2 medium cucumbers, peeled and sliced thinly
- 1/2 medium sweet onion, sliced
- 1/4 cup white wine vinegar
- 1 tablespoon canola oil
- 1/8 teaspoon black pepper
- 1/2 cup reduced-fat sour cream

DIRECTIONS:

1. Toss in cucumber, onion, and all other ingredients in a medium-size bowl.
2. Mix well and refrigerate for 2 hours.
3. Toss again and serve to enjoy.

Nutrition: *Calories: 64 Protein: 1g Carbohydrates: 4g Fat: 5g Cholesterol: 3mg Sodium: 72mg Potassium: 113mg Phosphorus: 24mg Calcium: 21mg Fiber: 0.8g*

CEREAL MUNCH

INGREDIENTS:

- 3 cups cereal, salt-free
- 1 ½ cups oyster crackers, salt-free
- 2 ½ tablespoons butter, unsalted
- ½ cup pretzel twists, salt-free
- ½ tablespoon chili powder
- 1 pinch ground cumin
- ¼ teaspoon garlic powder
- 1 pinch cayenne pepper
- ¾ teaspoons lemon juice

DIRECTIONS:

1. Brush a 10x15 inches pan with melted butter.
2. Toss the pretzels and crackers with the remaining ingredients in the baking tray.
3. Bake them for 45 minutes in the oven at 350 degrees F.
4. Toss the cereal munch every 15 minutes.
5. Serve.

Nutrition: *Calories: 379 Total Fat: 11.2g Saturated Fat: 1.8g Cholesterol: 0mg Sodium: 254mg Carbohydrate: 48.9g Dietary Fiber: 9.3g Sugars: 21.3g Protein: 8.3g Calcium: 28mg Phosphorous: 319mg Potassium: 365mg*

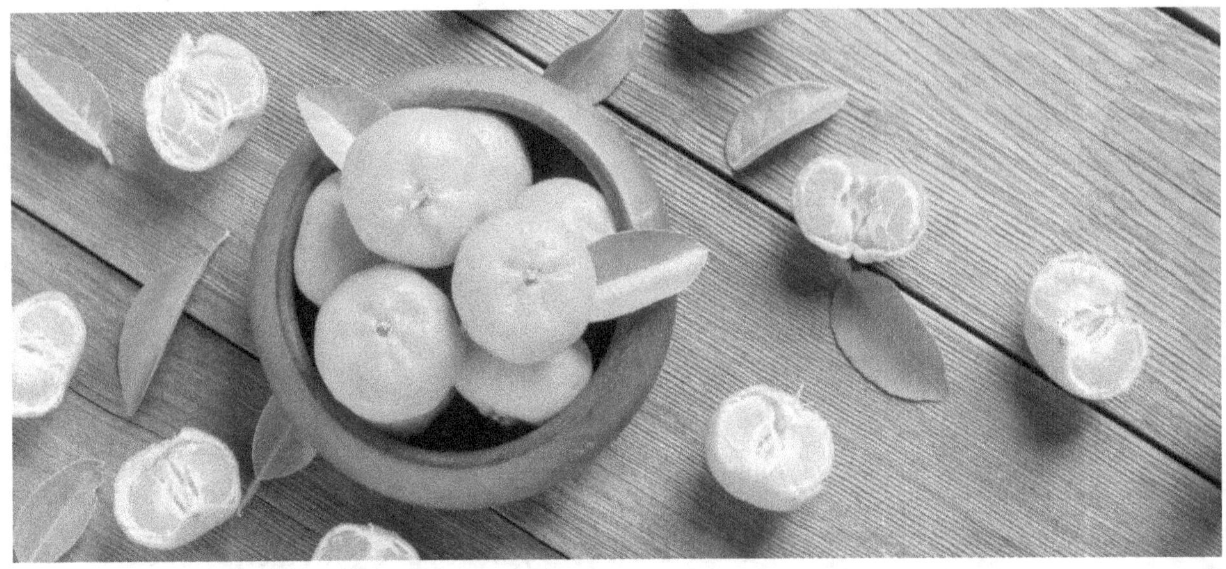

COCONUT MANDARIN SALAD

INGREDIENTS:

- 20 oz. can pineapple chunks
- 11 oz. canned mandarin oranges
- 10 oz. maraschino cherries, cut in halves
- 16 oz. sour cream
- 2 cups shredded sweetened coconut

DIRECTIONS:

1. Toss the pineapples with the cherries, oranges, coconut, and sour cream in a bowl.
2. Serve fresh.

Nutrition: *Calories: 372 Total Fat: 24.9g Saturated Fat: 17.8g Cholesterol: 33mg Sodium: 49mg Total Carbohydrate: 36.2g Dietary Fiber: 4.3g Sugars: 28.8g Protein: 3.9g Phosphorous: 356mg Potassium: 464mg*

CREAM DIPPED CUCUMBERS

INGREDIENTS:

- 1/2 cup sour cream
- 3 tablespoons white vinegar
- 1 teaspoon stevia
- Pepper to taste
- 4 cucumbers, peeled and sliced
- 1 small sweet onion, cut into rings

DIRECTIONS:

1. Use a medium-sized serving bowl.
2. Add in the cucumber, onion, and all the other ingredients.
3. Mix them well and refrigerate for 2 hours.
4. Toss again, serve and enjoy.

Nutrition: *Calories: 127 Total Fat: 6.4g Saturated Fat: 3.9g Cholesterol: 13mg Sodium: 23mg Carbohydrate: 9.2g Dietary Fiber: 1.9g Sugars: 4.2g Protein: 3.1g Calcium: 86mg Phosphorous: 172mg Potassium: 518mg*

BARBECUE CUPS

INGREDIENTS:

- ¾ lb. lean ground turkey
- ½ cup spicy barbecue sauce
- 2 teaspoons onion flakes
- 1 dash garlic powder
- 1 (10-oz.) package low-fat biscuits

DIRECTIONS:

1. Grease a suitable pan with cooking spray and place it over moderate heat.
2. Add the ground turkey and sauté it until golden brown.
3. Flatten the biscuits and place them in a muffin tray.
4. Press each biscuit in its muffin cup and divide the turkey in them.
5. Top the turkey with barbecue sauce, garlic powder, and onion flakes.
6. Bake for 12 minutes at 400 degrees F in a preheated oven.
7. Serve.

Nutrition: *Calories: 143 Total Fat: 6.3g Saturated Fat: 1.8g Cholesterol: 25mg Sodium: 329mg Carbohydrate: 13.1g Dietary Fiber: 0.2g Sugars: 2.7g Protein: 8.6g Calcium: 21mg Phosphorous: 367mg Potassium: 164mg*

SPICED PRETZELS

INGREDIENTS:

- 1 teaspoon ground cayenne pepper
- 1 teaspoon lemon pepper
- 1 1/2 teaspoons garlic powder
- 1 oz. dry Ranch-style dressing
- 3/4 cup vegetable oil
- 15 oz. packages mini pretzels

DIRECTIONS:

1. Switch the oven to 175 degrees F to preheat.
2. Spread the pretzels on a cooking sheet and break them into pieces.
3. Whisk the oil with the garlic powder, lemon pepper, ground cayenne pepper, and ranch dressing in a bowl.
4. Pour this oil dressing over the pretzels and toss well to coat.
5. Bake the pretzels for approximately 1 hour then flip them to bake for another 15 minutes.
6. Serve fresh and warm.

Nutrition: *Calories: 311 Total Fat: 18.6g Saturated Fat: 3.2g Cholesterol: 0mg Sodium: 270mg Carbohydrate: 33.2g Dietary Fiber: 1.6g Sugars: 0g Protein: 3g Calcium: 1mg Phosphorous: 371mg Potassium: 6mg*

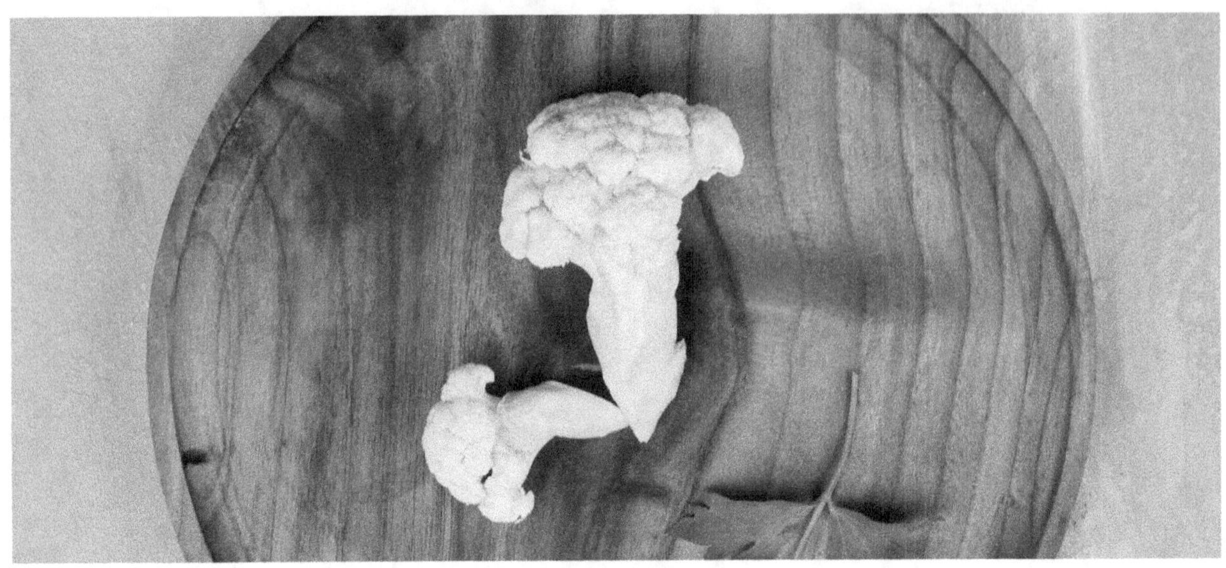

CAULIFLOWER
WITH MUSTARD SAUCE

INGREDIENTS:

- 1 head cauliflower, separated into florets
- 1/2 cup mayonnaise
- 1/4 cup Dijon mustard
- 1 cup sharp Cheddar cheese, shredded

DIRECTIONS:

1. Whisk the mayonnaise with the mustard and cheese in a bowl.
2. Add the cauliflower florets in boiling water in a pot and cook until they are tender.
3. Drain the cauliflower then toss its florets with the mayo mixture.
4. Spread the cauliflower mixture in a baking pan.
5. Broil it for 5 minutes until the cheese is melted.
6. Serve fresh.

Nutrition: *Calories: 255 Total Fat: 19.9g Saturated Fat: 7.5g Cholesterol: 37mg Sodium: 582mg Carbohydrate: 11.7g Dietary Fiber: 2.2g Sugars: 3.8g Protein: 9.3g Calcium: 231mg Phosphorous: 97mg Potassium: 253mg*

PINEAPPLE CABBAGE COLESLAW

INGREDIENTS:

- 12 oz. (bag) broccoli coleslaw
- 12 oz. Napa cabbage, finely shredded
- 20 oz. (can) unsweetened pineapple, drained
- 1/2 cup green onions, sliced
- 1 cup mayonnaise
- 1 tablespoon seasoned rice vinegar
- 1 teaspoon coarse ground black pepper

DIRECTIONS:

1. Toss the cabbage with the broccoli, and all the other ingredients in a salad bowl.
2. Refrigerate this coleslaw for at least 1 hour.
3. Serve.

Nutrition: *Calories: 186 Total Fat: 12.7g Saturated Fat: 2g Cholesterol: 5mg Sodium: 224mg Carbohydrate: 18g Dietary Fiber: 2.1g Sugars: 10.4g Protein: 2g Calcium: 42mg Phosphorous: 106mg Potassium: 139mg*

MASHED CAULIFLOWER

INGREDIENTS:

- 1 cauliflower head
- 1 tablespoon olive oil
- ½ tsp salt
- ¼ tsp dill
- Pepper to taste
- 2 tbsp low fat milk

DIRECTIONS:

1. Bring a small pot of water to a boil.
2. Chop cauliflower in florets.
3. Add florets to boiling water and boil uncovered for 5 minutes. Turn off the fire and let it sit for 5 minutes more.
4. In a blender, add all ingredients except for cauliflower and blend to mix well.
5. Drain cauliflower well and add into the blender. Puree until smooth and creamy.
6. Serve and enjoy.

Nutrition: *Calories: 78 Fat: 5g Carbs: 6g Protein: 2g Fiber: 2g Sodium: 420mg Potassium: 327mg*

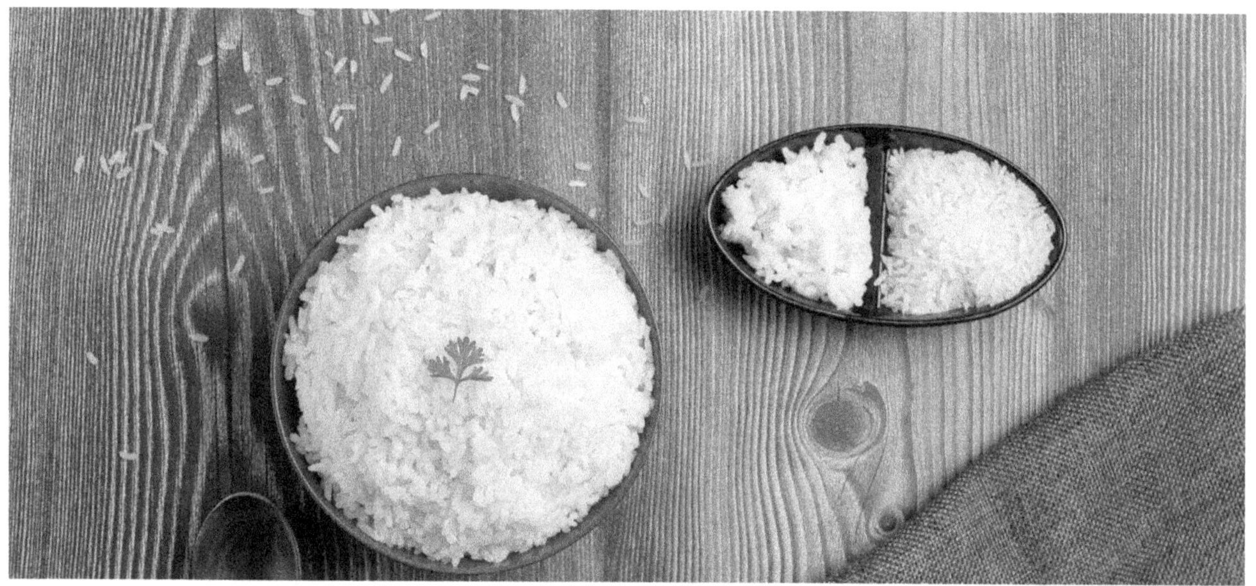

SWEET RICE SALAD

INGREDIENTS:

- 3 tablespoons apricot jam
- 1 tablespoon water
- 1 tablespoon lemon juice
- 7 tablespoons mayonnaise
- 6 oz. long-grain rice, cooked & rinsed
- 1 oz. onion, finely chopped
- 2 apples, chopped
- 8 cherry tomatoes

DIRECTIONS:

1. Mix the rice with the apples, tomatoes, and onion in a salad bowl.
2. Whisk the apricot jam and the rest of the dressing ingredients in a small bowl.
3. Pour this dressing into the rice salad and mix well.
4. Serve.

Nutrition: *Calories: 265 Total Fat: 6.4g Saturated Fat: 1g Cholesterol: 4mg Sodium: 137mg Carbohydrate: 49.2g Dietary Fiber: 4.3g Sugars: 17.8g Protein: 4g Calcium: 30mg Phosphorous: 258mg Potassium: 520mg*

HERBED SHRIMP SPREAD

INGREDIENTS:

- 1/2 lb. shrimp, cooked, peeled and deveined
- 1/2 cup reduced-fat sour cream
- 1/2 cup light mayonnaise
- 2 scallions, coarsely chopped
- 1 teaspoon lemon zest, finely grated
- 2 teaspoons fresh lemon juice
- 1/4 cup parsley, chopped

DIRECTIONS:

1. Begin by tossing the minced shrimp with the sour cream in a bowl.
2. Add in the mayonnaise, scallions, lemon juice and lemon zest.
3. Mix well and garnish with parsley.
4. Serve the spread.

Nutrition: *Calories: 118 Total Fat: 8.3g Saturated Fat: 2.7g Cholesterol: 65mg Sodium: 177mg Carbohydrate: 4.6g Dietary Fiber: 0.2g Sugars: 1.1g Protein: 6.7g Calcium: 35mg Phosphorous: 203mg Potassium: 95mg*

ALMOND CARAMEL

CORN

INGREDIENTS:

- 12 cups popped popcorn
- 3 cups unblanched whole almonds
- 1 cup brown Swerve
- ½ cup butter
- ¼ cup light corn syrup
- ½ teaspoon baking soda

DIRECTIONS:

1. Take a suitable roasting pan and spread the almonds and popcorn in it.
2. Whisk the Swerve with the butter and corn syrup in a heavy saucepan.
3. Stir-fry this corn syrup for about 5 minutes up to a boil then add in the baking soda.
4. Pour this corn sauce over the popcorn and almonds in the pan.
5. Bake the popcorn mixture for approximately 1 hour at 200 degrees F in the oven.
6. Stir well then serve.

Nutrition: *Calories: 120 Total Fat: 8g Saturated Fat: 2.3g Cholesterol: 8mg Sodium: 45mg Carbohydrate: 6.5g Dietary Fiber: 1.7g Sugars: 1.1g Protein: 2.5g Calcium: 31mg Phosphorous: 23mg Potassium: 88mg*

JALAPENO
TOMATO SALSA

INGREDIENTS:

- 4 jalapeños, seeded and chopped
- 3 garlic cloves, peeled
- 1/2 white onion, chopped
- 2 lb. tomatoes, quartered
- Juice of 1/2 lime

DIRECTIONS:

1. Add the jalapeños, garlic, onion, tomatoes, and lime juice into a blender.
2. Blend this salsa mixture until it gets chunky.
3. Serve fresh.

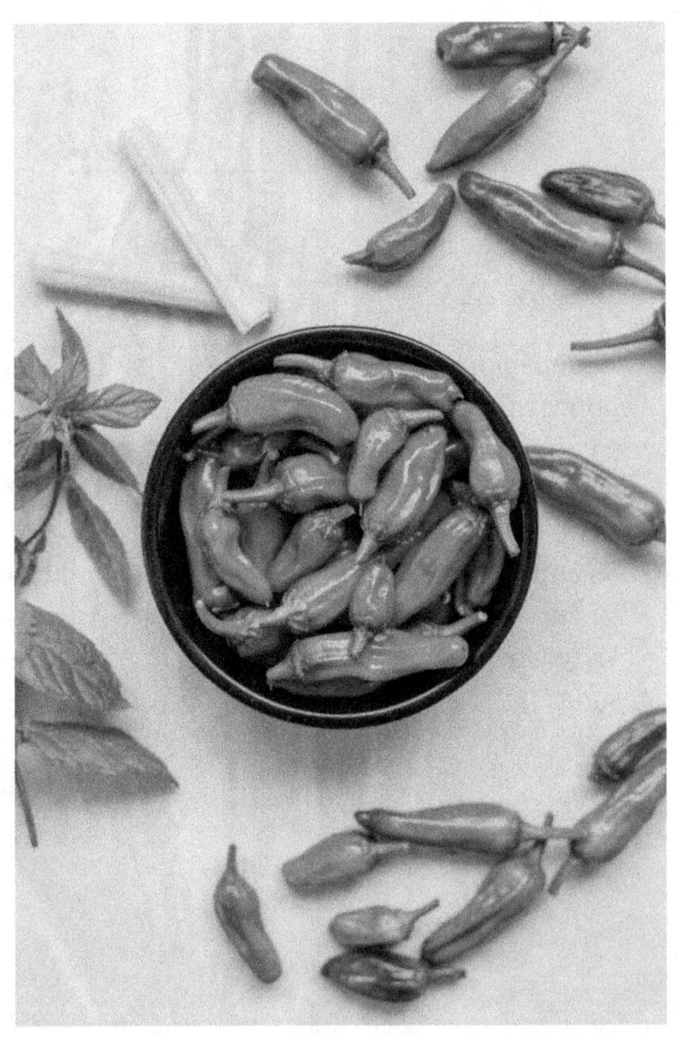

Nutrition: *Calories: 32 Total Fat: 0.3g Saturated Fat: 0g Cholesterol: 0mg Sodium: 638mg Carbohydrate: 5.3g Dietary Fiber: 1.6g Sugars: 3.2g Protein: 1.1g Calcium: 13mg Phosphorous: 33mg Potassium: 244mg*

CHAPTER 8

Dessert Recipes

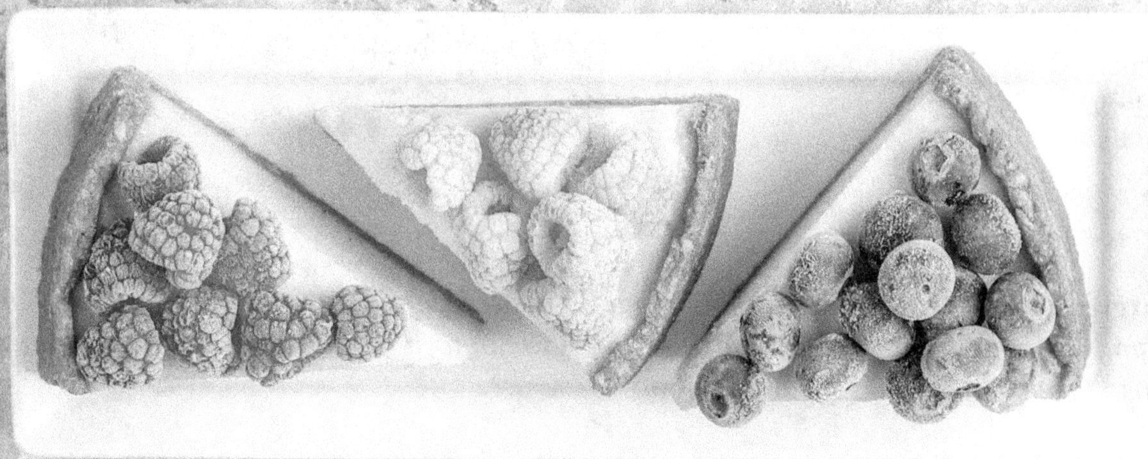

CHOCOLATE TRIFLE

INGREDIENTS:

- 1 small plain sponge swiss roll
- 3 oz. custard powder
- 5 oz. hot water
- 16 oz. canned mandarins
- 3 tablespoons sherry
- 5 oz. double cream
- 4 chocolate squares, grated

DIRECTIONS:

1. Whisk the custard powder with water in a bowl until dissolved.
2. In a bowl, mix the custard well until it becomes creamy and let it sit for 15 minutes.
3. Spread the swiss roll and cut it in 4 squares.
4. Place the swiss roll in the 4 serving cups.
5. Top the swiss roll with mandarin, custard, cream, and chocolate.
6. Serve.

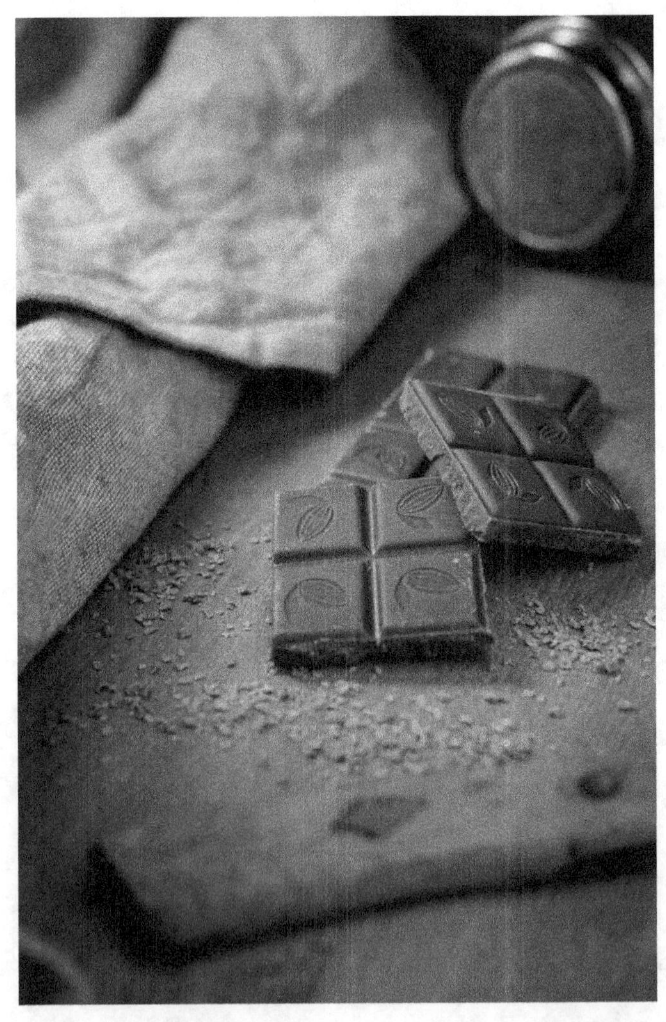

Nutrition: *Calories: 315 Total Fat: 13.5g Saturated Fat: 8.4g Cholesterol: 43mg Sodium: 185mg Carbohydrate: 40.1g Dietary Fiber: 1.4g Sugars: 9.1g Protein: 2.9g Calcium: 61mg Phosphorous: 184mg Potassium: 129mg*

PINEAPPLE MERINGUES

INGREDIENTS:

- 4 meringue nests
- 8 oz. crème fraiche
- 2 oz. stem ginger, chopped
- 8 oz. can pineapple chunks

DIRECTIONS:

1. Place the meringue nests on the serving plates.
2. Whisk the ginger with crème Fraiche and pineapple chunks.
3. Divide the pineapple mixture over the meringue nests.
4. Serve.

Nutrition: *Calories: 312 Total Fat: 22.8g Saturated Fat: 0g Cholesterol: 0mg Sodium: 41mg Carbohydrate: 25g Dietary Fiber: 0.7g Sugars: 23.1g Protein: 2.3g Calcium: 3mg Phosphorous: 104mg Potassium: 110mg*

BAKED CUSTARD

INGREDIENTS:

- 1/2 cup milk
- 1 egg, beaten
- 1/8 teaspoon nutmeg
- 1/8 teaspoon vanilla
- Sweetener, to taste
- 1/2 cup water

DIRECTIONS:

1. Lightly warm up the milk in a pan, then whisk in the egg, nutmeg, vanilla and sweetener.
2. Pour this custard mixture into a ramekin.
3. Place the ramekin in a baking pan and pour ½ cup water into the pan.
4. Bake the custard for 30 minutes at 325 degrees F.
5. Serve fresh.

Nutrition: *Calories: 127 Total Fat: 7g Saturated Fat: 2.9g Cholesterol: 174mg Sodium: 119mg Carbohydrate: 6.6g Dietary Fiber: 0.1g Sugars: 6g Protein: 9.6g Calcium: 169mg Phosphorous: 309mg Potassium: 171mg*

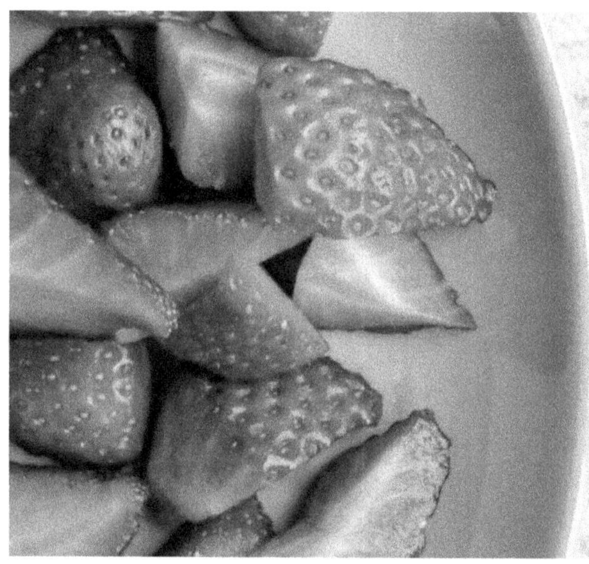 

STRAWBERRY PIE

INGREDIENTS:

- 1 unbaked (9 inches) pie shell
- 4 cups strawberries, fresh
- 1 cup of brown Swerve
- 3 tablespoons arrowroot powder
- 2 tablespoons lemon juice
- 8 tablespoons whipped cream topping

DIRECTIONS:

1. Spread the pie shell in the pie pan and bake it until golden brown.
2. Now mash 2 cups of strawberries with the lemon juice, arrowroot powder, and Swerve in a bowl.
3. Add the mixture to a saucepan and cook on moderate heat until it thickens.
4. Allow the mixture to cool then spread it in the pie shell.
5. Slice the remaining strawberries and spread them over the pie filling.
6. Refrigerate for 1 hour then garnish with whipped cream.
7. Serve fresh and enjoy.

Nutrition: *Calories: 236 Total Fat: 11.1g Saturated Fat: 3.3g Cholesterol: 3mg Sodium: 183mg Carbohydrate: 26g Dietary Fiber: 2.3g Sugars: 7.5g Protein: 2.2g Calcium: 23mg Phosphorous: 47.2mg Potassium: 178mg*

APPLE CRISP

INGREDIENTS:

- 4 cups apples, peeled and chopped
- ½ teaspoon stevia
- 3 tablespoons brandy
- 2 teaspoons lemon juice
- 1/2 teaspoon cinnamon
- 1/8 teaspoon nutmeg
- 3/4 cup dry oats
- 1/4 cup brown Swerve
- 2 tablespoons flour
- 2 tablespoons butter

DIRECTIONS:

1. Toss the oats with the flour, butter and brown Swerve in a bowl and keep it aside.
2. Whisk the remaining crisp ingredients in an 8-inch baking pan.
3. Spread the oats mixture over the crispy filling.
4. Bake it for 45 minutes at 350 degrees F in a preheated oven.
5. Slice and serve.

Nutrition: *Calories: 214 Total Fat: 4.8g Saturated Fat: 0.8g Cholesterol: 0mg Sodium: 48mg Carbohydrate: 26.2g Dietary Fiber: 4.8g Sugars: 15.7g Protein: 2.1g Calcium: 15mg Phosphorous: 348mg Potassium: 212mg*

ALMOND COOKIES

INGREDIENTS:

- 1 cup butter, softened
- 1 cup granulated Swerve
- 1 egg
- 3 cups flour
- 1 teaspoon baking soda
- 1 teaspoon almond extract

DIRECTIONS:

1. Beat the butter with the Swerve in a mixer then gradually stir in the remaining ingredients.
2. Mix well until it forms a cookie dough then divide the dough into small balls.
3. Spread each ball into ¾ inch rounds and place them on a cookie sheet.
4. Poke 2-3 holes in each cookie then bake for 12 minutes at 400 degrees F.
5. Serve.

Nutrition: *Calories 159 Total Fat 7.9g Saturated Fat 1.3g Cholesterol 7mg Sodium 144mg Carbohydrate 6.8g Dietary Fiber 0.4g Sugars 3.1g Protein 1.9g Calcium 6mg Phosphorous 274mg Potassium 23mg*

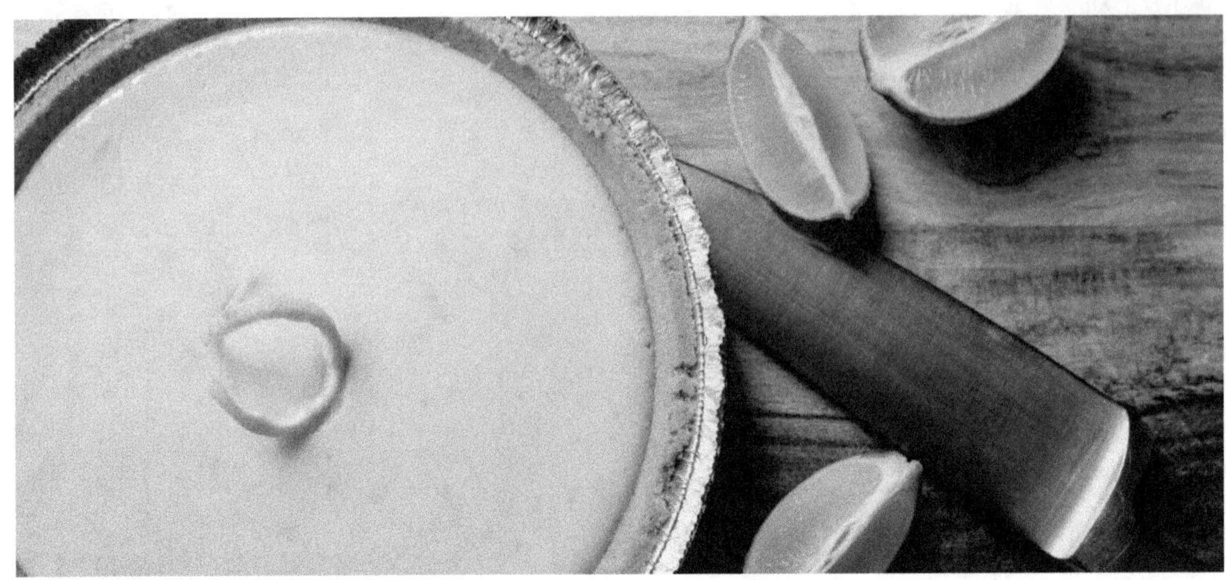

LIME PIE

INGREDIENTS:

- 5 tablespoons butter, unsalted
- 1 1/4 cups breadcrumbs
- 1/4 cup granulated Swerve
- 1/3 cup lime juice
- 14 oz. condensed milk
- 1 cup heavy whipping cream
- 1 (9 inches) pie shell

DIRECTIONS:

1. Switch on your gas oven and preheat it to 350 degrees F.
2. Whisk the cracker crumbs with the Swerve and melted butter in a suitable bowl.
3. Spread this cracker crumbs crust in a 9 inches pie shell and bake it for 5 minutes.
4. Meanwhile, mix the condensed milk with the lime juice in a bowl.
5. Whisk the heavy cream in a mixer until foamy, then add in the condensed milk mixture.
6. Mix well, then spread this filling in the baked crust.
7. Refrigerate the pie for 4 hours.
8. Slice and serve.

Nutrition:*Calories: 391 Total Fat: 22.4g Saturated Fat: 11.5g Cholesterol: 57mg Sodium: 252mg Total Carbohydrate: 32.9g Dietary Fiber: 0.3g Sugars: 27.4g Protein: 5.3g Calcium: 163mg Phosphorous: 199mg Potassium: 221mg*

EASY TURNIP PUREE

INGREDIENTS:

- 1 1/2 lbs. turnips, peeled and chopped
- 1 tsp dill
- 3 bacon slices, cooked and chopped
- 2 tbsp fresh chives, chopped

DIRECTIONS:

1. Add turnip into the boiling water and cook for 12 minutes. Drain well and place in a food processor.
2. Add dill and process until smooth.
3. Transfer turnip puree into the bowl and top with bacon and chives.
4. Serve and enjoy.

Nutrition: *Calories: 127 Fat: 6g Carbohydrates: 11.6g Sugar: 7g Protein: 6.8g Cholesterol: 16mg*

VERY BERRY

BREAD PUDDING

INGREDIENTS:

- 8 cups cubed challah bread
- 6 eggs, beaten
- 2 cups heavy cream
- 12-ounce bag of frozen berry medley, thawed
- ½ cup sugar
- 2 teaspoons vanilla
- 1 tablespoon orange zest
- ½ teaspoon cinnamon
- Whipped cream

DIRECTIONS:

1. Preheat the oven to 375° F.
2. Beat eggs, sugar, cream, orange zest, vanilla and cinnamon until smooth.
3. Mix in bread cubes and fruit with hands.
4. Pour into buttered/greased pan and bake covered in foil for 35 minutes. If using butter, make sure it is unsalted.
5. Remove foil and bake for 15 additional minutes.
6. Turn off the oven and let sit in the oven for 10 minutes.
7. Cut, then serve topped with whipped cream.

TIPS: Serve as a special breakfast treat or for holiday brunch. If you wish to store or make it ahead of time, Very Berry Bread Pudding can be frozen until ready to thaw and reheat.

Nutrition: *Calories: 392kcal Total Fat: 23g Saturated Fat: 12g Cholesterol: 189g Sodium: 231mg Total Carbs: 36g Fiber: 2.2g Sugar: 0g Protein: 9g*

SUNBURST LEMON BARS

INGREDIENTS:

Crust:

- 2 cups all-purpose flour
- ½ cup powdered sugar
- 1 cup butter (2 sticks), unsalted, room temperature

Filling:

- 4 eggs
- 1½ cups sugar
- ¼ cup all-purpose flour
- ½ teaspoon cream of tartar
- ¼ teaspoon baking soda
- ¼ cup lemon juice

Glaze:

- 1 cup powdered sugar, sifted
- 2 tablespoons lemon juice

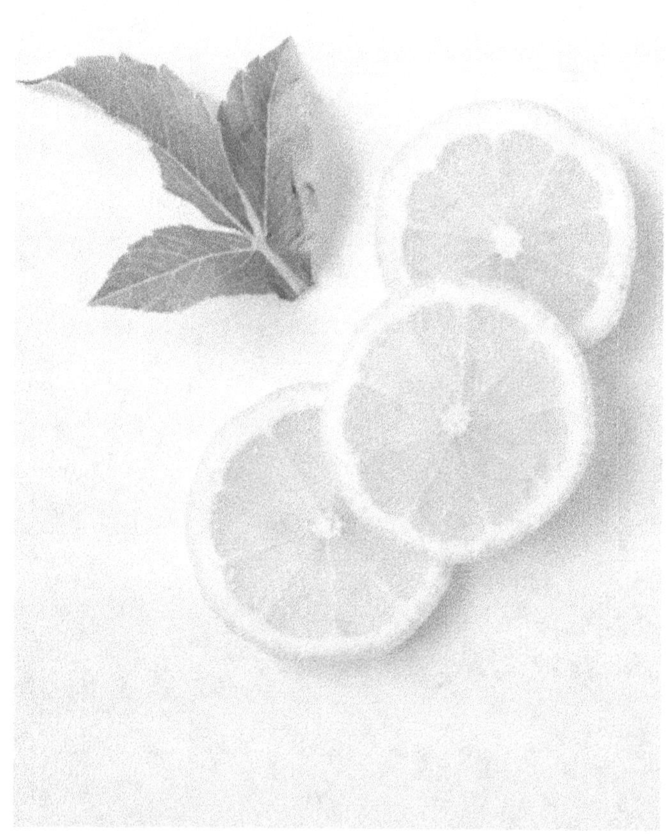

DIRECTIONS:

Crust:

1. Preheat oven to 350° F.
2. In a large bowl, combine the flour, powdered sugar and 1 cup of softened butter. Mix until crumbly. Press the mixture into the bottom of a 9" x 13" baking pan.
3. Bake until lightly browned, about 15–20 minutes.

Filling:

1. In a medium-sized bowl, whisk the eggs slightly.
2. In another bowl, combine the sugar, flour, cream of tartar and baking soda. Add the dry mixture to

the eggs. Add the lemon juice to the egg mixture and whisk until slightly thickened.

3. Pour over the warm crust and bake for another 20 minutes or until filling is set.

4. Remove from the oven and cool.

Glaze:

1. In a small bowl, gradually stir the lemon juice into the sifted powdered sugar until spreadable. Add more or less lemon juice as needed.

2. Spread over the cooled filling. Let the glaze set and then cut into 24 bars. Store extra lemon bars in the refrigerator.

Nutrition: *Calories: 200kcal Total Fat: 9g Saturated Fat: 5g Cholesterol: 53mg Sodium: 27mg Total Carbs: 28g Fiber: 0.3g Sugar: 0g Protein: 2g*

MOLTEN MINT CHOCOLATE BROWNIES

INGREDIENTS:

- 1 box Betty Crocker® brownie mix (not supreme)
- 12 Andes® mint chocolates
- Optional garnish: powdered sugar, cocoa powder (unsweetened or sweetened), fresh mint sprigs

DIRECTIONS:

1. Preheat oven and prepare brownie mixture according to the directions on the box.
2. Prepare 12 cup muffin tin with liner or lightly grease and flour the bottom and sides. Pour the brownie mix into the pans and bake for 25 minutes.
3. Remove brownies from oven and insert one piece of mint candy in the center and bake for an additional 5 minutes. Turn off the oven and remove. Let cool for 5–10 minutes.
4. Remove brownie cupcakes from pan and then serve.

Nutrition: *Calories: 307kcal Total Fat: 18g Saturated Fat: 4g Cholesterol: 32mg Sodium: 147mg Total Carbs: 36g Fiber: 0g Sugar: 0g Protein: 3g*

FESTIVE CREAM CHEESE SUGAR COOKIES

INGREDIENTS:

- 1 cup sugar
- 1 cup butter, unsalted, softened
- 3 ounces cream cheese, softened
- 1 large egg, separated
- ½ teaspoon salt
- ¼ teaspoon almond extract
- ½ teaspoon vanilla extract
- 2¼ cups all-purpose flour
- Optional garnish: colored sugar

DIRECTIONS:

1. In a large bowl, combine sugar, butter, cream cheese, salt, almond extract, vanilla extract and egg yolk. Blend well. Stir in flour until well-blended.
2. Chill cookie dough for 2 hours in the refrigerator.
3. Preheat oven to 350° F.
4. On a lightly floured surface, roll out the dough, one third at a time to ¼–inch thickness. Cut into desired shapes with lightly floured cookie cutters.
5. Place them 1 inch apart on ungreased cookie sheets. Leave cookies plain, or if desired, brush with slightly beaten egg white and sprinkle with colored sugar.
6. Bake cream cheese cookies for 7–9 minutes or until light golden brown. Let cool completely before serving.

Nutrition: *Calories: 79kcal Total Fat: 5g Saturated Fat: 3g Cholesterol: 16mg Sodium: 33mg Total Carbs: 0g Fiber: 0g Sugar: 0g Protein: 1g*

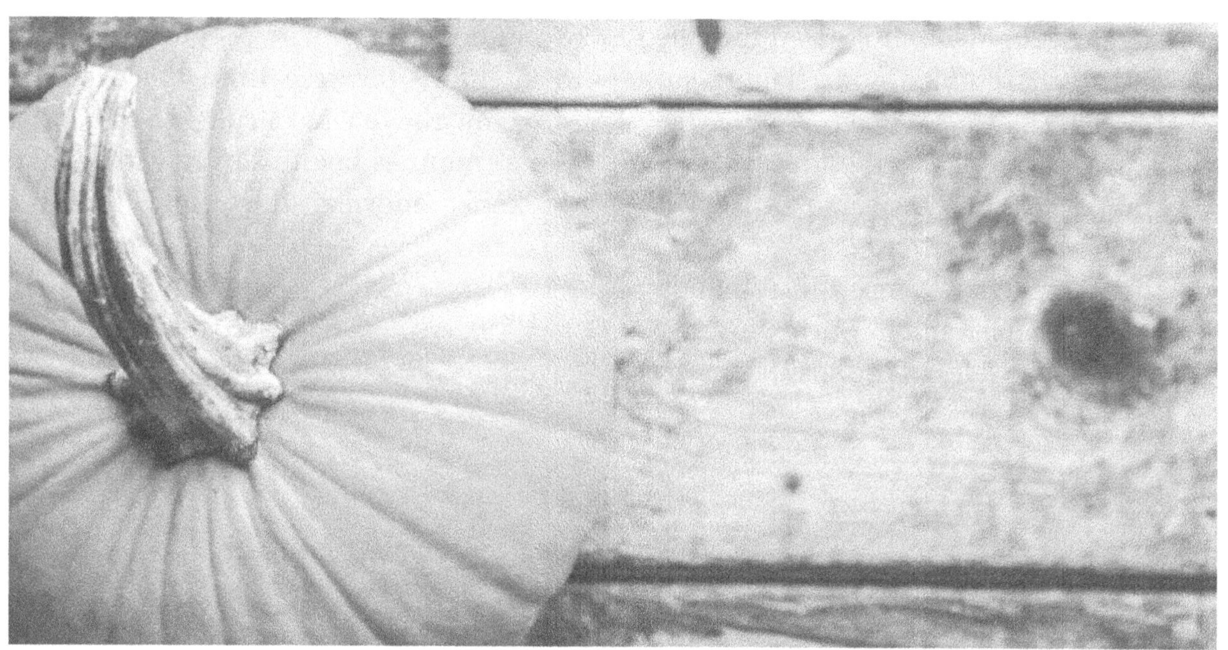

PUMPKIN STRUDEL

INGREDIENTS:

- 1½ cups canned pumpkin, sodium-free, unsweetened
- ⅛ teaspoon grated nutmeg
- 1 teaspoon pure vanilla extract
- 4 tablespoons sugar

- ½ teaspoon ground cinnamon
- ½ stick (4 tablespoons) butter, unsalted, melted
- 12 sheets phyllo dough (follow package directions for defrosting if frozen)

DIRECTIONS:

1. Position the oven rack in the middle of the oven. Preheat the oven to 375° F.
2. In a medium-sized bowl, combine the canned pumpkin, nutmeg, vanilla extract, 2 tablespoons of sugar and ½ tablespoon of cinnamon until well-mixed.
3. Using a pastry brush, coat the bottom of a nonstick medium sheet tray with the melted butter. On a clean work surface, lay down a single sheet of phyllo dough, and brush it with the butter. Then create a stack of buttered phyllo sheets, brushing every other phyllo sheet with butter. (Be sure to save a little melted butter to brush the top of the rolled filled strudel, so go lightly when brushing in between layers.) Keep remaining phyllo dough sheets covered with plastic wrap until ready for use, so they do not dry out.

4. Once all 12 sheets are used, spoon the mixture evenly along one of the long edges of the stack. Roll from the filled end to the unfilled end, making sure the seam side faces down.

5. Transfer the roll to the greased sheet tray seam-side down and brush with the remaining butter.

6. In a small bowl, mix the remaining sugar and cinnamon. Sprinkle it over the top and sides of the strudel.

7. Bake on the middle rack until lightly toasted or golden brown, about 12–15 minutes.

8. Remove the tray from the oven and allow the toasted strudel to rest for 5–10 minutes before slicing with a sharp knife, allowing the center to settle. Serve.

Nutrition: *Calories: 180kcal Total Fat: 8g Saturated Fat: 4g Cholesterol: 16mg Sodium: 41mg Total Carbs: 0g Fiber: 0g Sugar: 0g Protein: 3g*

PREPARATION: 5 MIN   **COOKING:** 10 MIN   **SERVINGS:** 2

SPICED PEACHES

INGREDIENTS:

- Canned peaches with juices – 1 cup
- Cornstarch – ½ tsp.
- Ground cloves – 1 tsp.
- Ground cinnamon – 1 tsp.
- Ground nutmeg – 1 tsp.
- Zest of ½ lemon
- Water – ½ cup

DIRECTIONS:

1. Drain peaches.
2. Combine cinnamon, cornstarch, nutmeg, ground cloves, and lemon zest in a pan on the stove.
3. Heat on medium heat and add peaches.
4. Bring to a boil, reduce the heat and simmer for 10 minutes.
5. Serve.

Nutrition: *Calories: 70kcal Total Fat: 0g Saturated Fat: 0g Cholesterol: 0mg Sodium: 3mg Total Carbs: 14g Fiber: 0g Sugar: 0g Protein: 1g*

PUMPKIN

CHEESECAKE BAR

INGREDIENTS:

- Unsalted butter – 2 ½ Tbsps.
- Cream cheese – 4 oz.
- All-purpose white flour – ½ cup
- Golden brown sugar – 3 Tbsps.
- Granulated sugar – ¼ cup
- Pureed pumpkin – ½ cup
- Egg whites – 2
- Ground cinnamon – 1 tsp.
- Ground nutmeg – 1 sp.
- Vanilla extract – 1 tsp.

DIRECTIONS:

1. Preheat the oven to 350F.
2. Mix flour and brown sugar in a bowl.
3. Mix in the butter to form 'breadcrumbs.'
4. Place ¾ of this mixture in a dish.
5. Bake in the oven for 15 minutes. Remove and cool.
6. Lightly whisk the egg and fold in the cream cheese, sugar, pumpkin, cinnamon, nutmeg and vanilla until smooth.
7. Pour this mixture over the oven-baked base and sprinkle with the rest of the breadcrumbs from earlier.
8. Bake in the oven for 30 to 35 minutes more.
9. Cool, slice and serve.

Nutrition: *Calories: 248kcal Total Fat: 13g Saturated Fat: 0g Cholesterol: 0mg Sodium: 146mg Total Carbs: 33g Fiber: 0g Sugar: 0g Protein: 4g*

BLUEBERRY MINI MUFFINS

INGREDIENTS:

- Egg whites – 3
- All-purpose white flour – ¼ cup
- Coconut flour – 1 Tbsp.
- Baking soda – 1 tsp.
- Nutmeg – 1 Tbsp. grated
- Vanilla extract – 1 tsp.
- Stevia – 1 tsp.
- Fresh blueberries – ¼ cup

DIRECTIONS:

1. Preheat the oven to 325°F.
2. Mix all the ingredients in a bowl.
3. Divide the batter into 4 and spoon into a lightly oiled muffin tin.
4. Bake in the oven for 15 to 20 minutes or until cooked through.
5. Cool and serve.

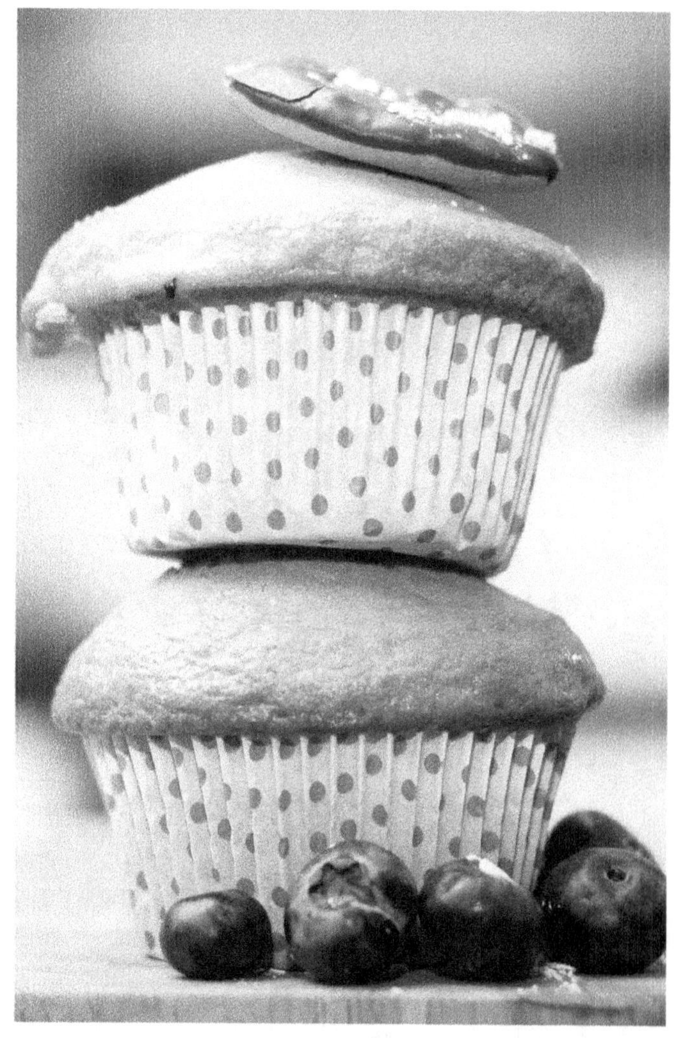

Nutrition: *Calories: 62kcal Total Fat: 0g Saturated Fat: 0g Cholesterol: 0mg Sodium: 62mg Total Carbs: 9g Fiber: 0g Sugar: 0g Protein: 4g*

VANILLA CUSTARD

INGREDIENTS:

- Egg – 1
- Vanilla – 1/8 tsp.
- Nutmeg – 1/8 tsp.
- Almond milk – ½ cup
- Stevia – 2 Tbsp.

DIRECTIONS:

1. Scald the milk then let it cool slightly.
2. Break the egg into a bowl and beat it with the nutmeg.
3. Add the scalded milk, the vanilla, and the sweetener to taste. Mix well.
4. Place the bowl in a baking pan filled with ½ deep of water.
5. Bake for 30 minutes at 325°F.
6. Serve.

Nutrition: *Calories: 167.3kcal Total Fat: 9g Saturated Fat: 0g Cholesterol: 0mg Sodium: 124mg Total Carbs: 11g Fiber: 0g Sugar: 0g Protein: 10g*

CHOCOLATE

CHIP COOKIES

INGREDIENTS:

- Semi-sweet chocolate chips – ½ cup
- Baking soda – ½ tsp.
- Vanilla – ½ tsp.
- Egg – 1
- Flour – 1 cup
- Margarine – ½ cup
- Stevia – 4 tsp.

DIRECTIONS:

1. Sift the dry ingredients.
2. Cream the margarine, stevia, vanilla and egg with a whisk.
3. Add flour mixture and beat well.
4. Stir in the chocolate chips, then drop teaspoonfuls of the mixture over a greased baking sheet.
5. Bake the cookies for about 10 minutes at 375°F.
6. Cool and serve.

Nutrition: *Calories: 106.2kcal Total Fat: 7g Saturated Fat: 0g Cholesterol: 0mg Sodium: 98mg Total Carbs: 8.9g Fiber: 0g Sugar: 0g Protein: 1.5g*

BAKED PEACHES
WITH CREAM CHEESE

INGREDIENTS:

- Plain cream cheese – 1 cup
- Crushed meringue cookies – ½ cup
- Ground cinnamon – ¼ tsp.
- Pinch ground nutmeg
- Canned peach halves – 8, in juice
- Honey – 2 Tbsp.

DIRECTIONS:

1. Preheat the oven to 350°F.
2. Line a baking sheet with parchment paper. Set aside.
3. In a small bowl, stir together the meringue cookies, cream cheese, cinnamon, and nutmeg.
4. Spoon the cream cheese mixture evenly into the cavities in the peach halves.
5. Place the peaches on the baking sheet and bake for 15 minutes or until the fruit is soft and the cheese is melted.
6. Remove the peaches from the baking sheet onto plates.
7. Drizzle with honey and serve.

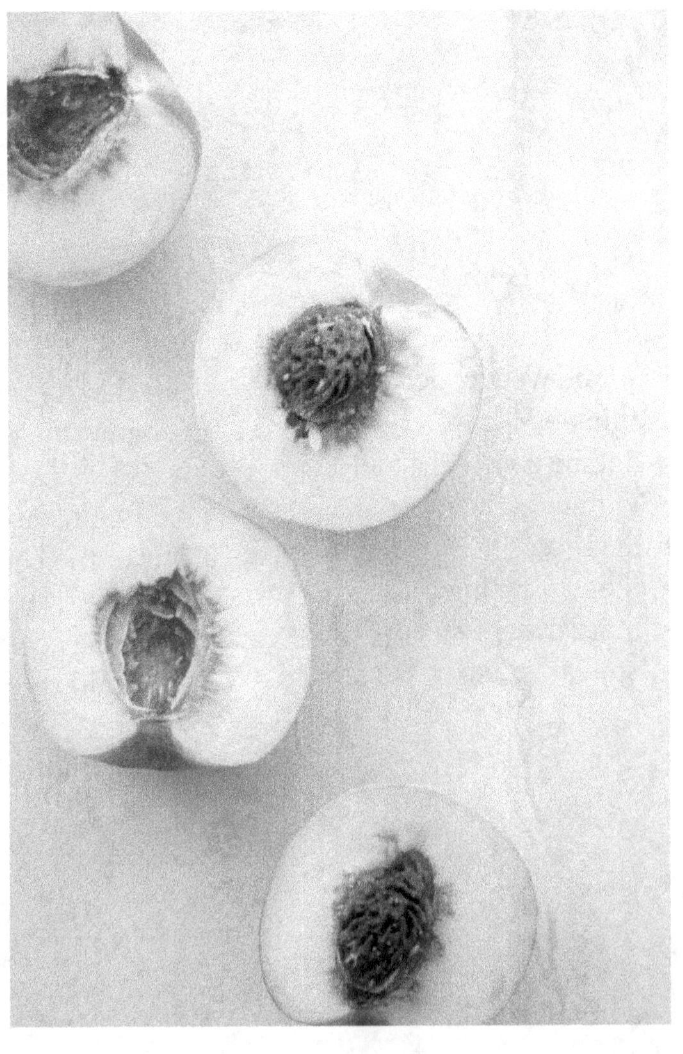

Nutrition: *Calories: 260kcal Total Fat: 20g Saturated Fat: 0g Cholesterol: 0mg Sodium: 216mg Total Carbs: 19g Fiber: 0g Sugar: 0g Protein: 4g*

CAULIFLOWER

BAGEL

INGREDIENTS:

- 1 large cauliflower, divided into florets and roughly chopped
- ¼ cup nutritional yeast
- ¼ cup almond flour
- ½ teaspoon garlic powder
- 1 ½ teaspoon fine sea salt
- 2 whole eggs
- 1 tablespoon sesame seeds

DIRECTIONS:

1. Preheat your oven to 400 °F.
2. Line a baking sheet with parchment paper, keep it on the side.
3. Blend cauliflower in a food processor and transfer to a bowl.
4. Add nutritional yeast, almond flour, garlic powder and salt to a bowl, mix.
5. Take another bowl and whisk in eggs, add to cauliflower mix.
6. Give the dough a stir.
7. Incorporate the mix into the egg mix.
8. Make balls from the dough, making a hole using your thumb into each ball.
9. Arrange them on your prepped sheet, flattening them into bagel shapes.
10. Sprinkle sesame seeds and bake for half an hour.
11. Remove the oven and let them cool, enjoy!

Nutrition: *Calories: 152 Fat: 10g Carbohydrates: 4g Protein: 4g*

STRAWBERRY

ICE CREAM

INGREDIENTS:

- Stevia – ½ cup
- Lemon juice – 1 Tbsp.
- Non-dairy coffee creamer – ¾ cup
- Strawberries – 10 oz.
- Crushed ice – 1 cup

DIRECTIONS:

1. Blend everything in a blend until smooth.
2. Freeze until frozen.
3. Serve.

Nutrition: *Calories: 94.4kcal Total Fat: 6g Saturated Fat: 0g Cholesterol: 0mg Sodium: 25mg Total Carbs: 8.3g Fiber: 0g Sugar: 0g Protein: 1.3g*

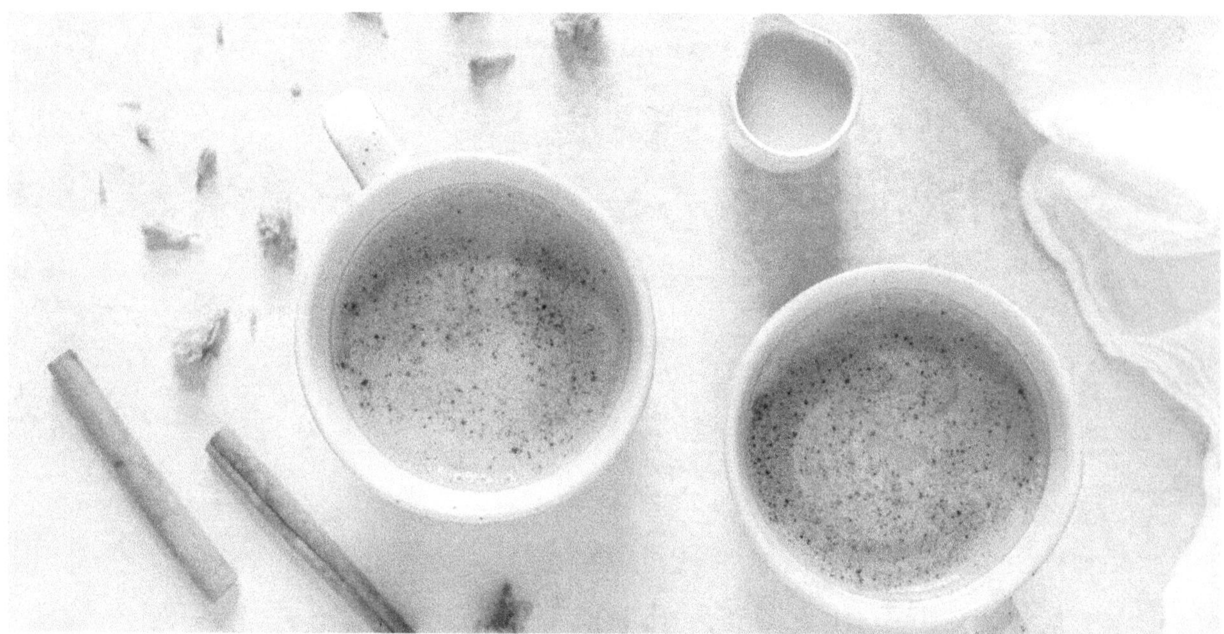

CINNAMON CUSTARD

INGREDIENTS:

- Unsalted butter, for greasing the ramekins
- Plain rice milk – 1 ½ cups
- Eggs – 4
- Granulated sugar – ¼ cup
- Pure vanilla extract – 1 tsp.
- Ground cinnamon – ½ tsp.
- Cinnamon sticks for garnish

DIRECTIONS:

1. Preheat the oven to 325°F.
2. Lightly grease 6 ramekins and place them in a baking dish. Set aside.
3. In a large bowl, whisk together the eggs, rice milk, sugar, vanilla, and cinnamon until the mixture is very smooth.
4. Pour the mixture through a fine sieve into a pitcher.
5. Evenly divide the custard mixture among the ramekins.
6. Fill the baking dish with hot water, until the water reaches halfway up the sides of the ramekins.
7. Bake for 1 hour or until the custards are set and a knife inserted in the center comes out clean.
8. Remove the custards from the oven and take the ramekins out of the water.
9. Cool on the wire racks for 1 hour then chill for 1 hour.
10. Garnish with cinnamon sticks and serve.

Nutrition: *Calories: 110kcal Total Fat: 4g Saturated Fat: 0g Cholesterol: 0mg Sodium: 71mg Total Carbs: 0g Fiber: 0g Sugar: 0g Protein: 4g*

ALMOND BITES

INGREDIENTS:

- 1/2 cup almond meal
- 2 tbsp coconut butter
- 4 dates, pitted and chopped
- 1/4 cup unsweetened chocolate chips
- 1 1/2 tsp vanilla

DIRECTIONS:

1. Add dates in the food processor and process for 30 seconds.
2. Add remaining ingredients except chocolate chips and process until combined.
3. Add chocolate chips and process for 15 seconds.
4. Make small balls from mixture and place on a baking tray.
5. Place in refrigerator for 1-2 hours.
6. Serve and enjoy

Nutrition: *Calories 53 Fat: 3.8g Carbohydrates: 4.2gSugar: 2.2g Protein: 1.1g Cholesterol: 1mg*

CHOCOLATE

COOKIES

INGREDIENTS:

- 2 eggs, lightly beaten
- 3 tbsp butter
- 3 tbsp unsweetened cocoa powder
- 1 1/2 cups almond flour
- 1 tsp vanilla
- 1/4 cup Swerve
- 3 oz unsweetened chocolate, chopped
- Pinch of salt

DIRECTIONS:

1. Add chocolate, butter, and cocoa powder into the pan and melt over medium-low heat.
2. Remove from heat and set aside.
3. Add eggs, vanilla, salt, and swerve in a bowl and blend until well combined.
4. Add melted chocolate mixture into the egg mixture and mix well.
5. Add almond flour and mix until well combined. Place in refrigerator for 1 hour.
6. Preheat the oven to 325F. Line baking tray with parchment paper and spray with cooking spray.
7. Scoop out batter onto a baking tray and bake for 10 minutes.
8. Serve and enjoy.

Nutrition: *Calories: 66 Fat: 5g Carbohydrates: 4.9g Sugar: 3g Protein: 2g Cholesterol: 25mg*

CHOCOLATE MUFFINS

INGREDIENTS:

- 2 eggs, lightly beaten
- 1/2 cup cream
- 1/2 tsp vanilla
- 1 cup almond flour
- 1 tbsp baking powder, gluten-free
- 4 tbsp Swerve
- 1/2 cup unsweetened cocoa powder
- Pinch of salt

DIRECTIONS:

1. Preheat the oven to 375F.
2. Spray a muffin tray with cooking spray and set aside.
3. In a mixing bowl, mix together almond flour, baking powder, swerve, cocoa powder, and salt.
4. In a separate bowl, beat eggs with cream, and vanilla.
5. Pour egg mixture into the almond flour mixture and mix well.
6. Pour batter into the prepared muffin tray and bake in preheated oven for 30 minutes.
7. Serve and enjoy.

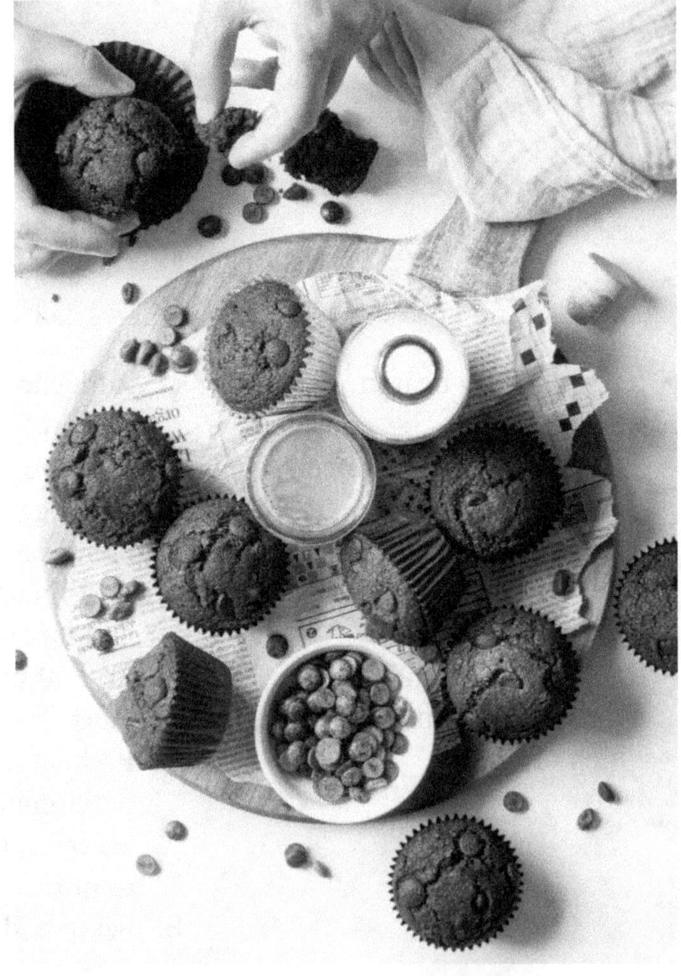

Nutrition: *Calories: 101 Fat: 7.5g Carbohydrates: 6.7g Sugar: 0.4g Protein: 4.5g Cholesterol: 35mg*

SWEET RASPBERRY

CANDY

INGREDIENTS:

- 1/2 cup dried raspberries
- 3 tbsp Swerve
- 1/2 cup coconut oil
- 2 oz cacao butter
- 1/2 tsp vanilla

DIRECTIONS:

1. Add cacao butter and coconut oil in a saucepan and melt over low heat. Remove from heat.
2. Grind the raspberries in a food processor.
3. Add sweetener and ground raspberries into the melted butter and coconut oil mixture and stir well.
4. Pour mixture into the mini silicone candy molds and place them in the refrigerator until set.
5. Serve and enjoy.

Nutrition: *Calories 103 Fat 11.5 g Carbohydrates 1.1 g Sugar 0.3 gProtein 0.1 g Cholesterol 0 mg*

INSTANT POT CHEESECAKE

INGREDIENTS:

- Graham Cracker Crust:
- 3 tablespoons sugar
- 5 tablespoons unsalted butter
- 9 large graham crackers, pulsed into crumbs
- 2 tablespoons ground pecans
- 1/4 teaspoons cinnamon
- Cheesecake Filling:
- 12 oz. cream cheese
- 2 teaspoons lemon zest
- 2 teaspoons vanilla extract
- 1 tablespoon cornstarch
- 1/2 cup + 2 tablespoons granulated sugar
- 2 large eggs + 1 egg yolk
- 1/2 cup sour cream

DIRECTIONS:

1. Start by heating sugar with butter in the microwave for 40 seconds.
2. Blend this melt with the cinnamon, pecan, and crumbs in a food processor.
3. Spread this mixture at the bottom of a baking pan.
4. Place this crust in the freezer for 1 hour.
5. Meanwhile, prepare the filling by beating all of its ingredients in an electric mixer.
6. Spread this filling into the prepared crust evenly.
7. Pour 2 cups water into the Instant Pot and place the steam rack over it.
8. Place the baking pan over the rack and seal the lid.
9. Select Manual mode with high pressure for 37 minutes.
10. Once the cooking is done, naturally release the pressure and remove the lid after 25 minutes.
11. Allow it to cool then remove the pie from the pan.
12. Refrigerate for 3 hours at minimum.
13. Slice and serve.

Nutrition: *Calories 177 Total Fats 9 g Saturated Fat 8.5 g Cholesterol 21 mg Sodium 95 mg Total Carbs 21 g Fiber 1.0 g Sugar 2.3 g Protein 3g*

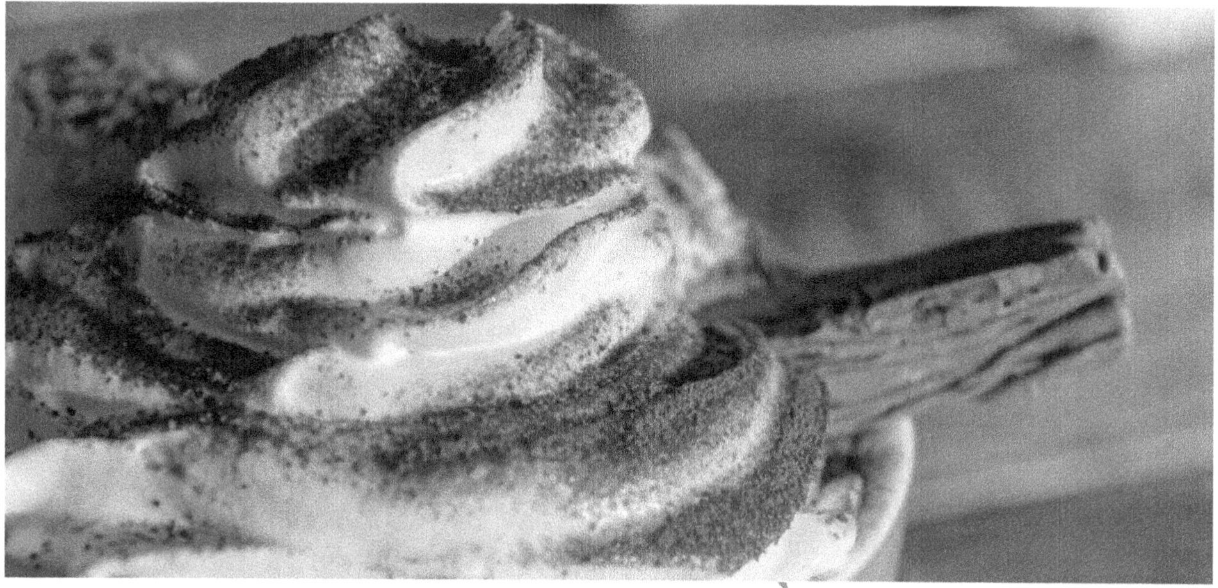

POTS DE CRÈME

INGREDIENTS:

- 1 1/2 cups heavy cream
- 1/2 cup coconut milk
- 5 large egg yolks
- 1/4 cup sugar
- 8 oz. bittersweet chocolate, melted
- Whipped cream and grated chocolate, to garnish

DIRECTIONS:

1. Start by heating cream with milk in a saucepan to a simmer.
2. Meanwhile, beat eggs yolks with sugar in a bowl.
3. Slowly pour in the hot milk mixture whiles stirring continuously.
4. Add chocolate and mix until fully incorporated.
5. Divide this mixture into 6 custard cups of equal size.
6. Pour 1.5 cups water into the Instant Pot and place the double steam rack over it.
7. Place the 3 custard cups over one rack and other 3 on the top rack.
8. Seal the pot's lid and cook for 6 minutes on Manual mode with High pressure.
9. Once the cooking is done, release the pressure completely then remove the lid.
10. Refrigerate the cups for 4 hours or more.
11. Serve.

Nutrition: *Calories 204 Total Fats8 g Saturated Fat 5.1 g Cholesterol 43 mg Sodium 113 mg Total Carbs 30 g Fiber 0.5 g Sugar 1.2 g Protein 3 g*

INGREDIENT CHEESECAKE

INGREDIENTS:

- Date and Nut Crust:
- 1 cup nuts
- 5 dates, roughly chopped
- Oatmeal Cookie Crust:
- ½ cup rolled oats
- ¼ cup pecans
- ¼ cup brown sugar
- 3 tablespoons melted butter
- Ingredient Cheesecake:
- 1 (14 ounces) can coconut milk with cream
- 1 cup yogurt
- Oil or butter, for greasing ramekins or cheesecake pan

DIRECTIONS:

1. Start by mixing the yogurt with the milk in a bowl.
2. Divide this mixture into 4 four ramekins, greased with cooking oil.
3. Place these ramekins in a baking pan.
4. After pouring 2 cups water into the Instant Pot, place the steam rack over it.
5. Cover the ramekins with aluminum foil and place the baking pan over the rack.
6. Seal the pot's lid and cook for 25 minutes on Manual mode with high pressure.
7. Once the cooking is done, release the pressure completely then remove the lid.
8. Allow the ramekins to cool at room temperature.
9. Refrigerate them for 6 hours.
10. Garnish as desired.
11. Serve.

Nutrition: *Calories 258 Total Fats 13 g Saturated Fat 9.1 g Cholesterol 11 mg Sodium 214 mg Total Carbs 28 g Fiber 1.0 g Sugar 1.3 g Protein 5 g*

RASPBERRY BRÛLÉE

INGREDIENTS:

- Light sour cream – ½ cup
- Plain cream cheese – ½ cup
- Brown sugar – ¼ cup, divided
- Ground cinnamon – ¼ tsp.
- Fresh raspberries – 1 cup

DIRECTIONS:

1. Preheat the oven to broil.
2. In a bowl, beat together the cream cheese, sour cream, 2 tbsp. brown sugar and cinnamon for 4 minutes or until the mixture is very smooth and fluffy.
3. Evenly divide the raspberries among 4 (4-ounce) ramekins.
4. Spoon the cream cheese mixture over the berries and smooth the tops.
5. Sprinkle ½ tbsp. brown sugar evenly over each ramekin.
6. Place the ramekins on a baking sheet and broil 4 inches from the heating element until the sugar is caramelized and golden brown.
7. Cool and serve.

Nutrition: *Calories: 188 kcal Total Fat: 13 g Saturated Fat: 0 g Cholesterol: 0 mg Sodium: 132 mg Total Carbs: 16 g Fiber: 0 g Sugar: 0 g Protein: 3 g*

GUMDROP COOKIES

INGREDIENTS:

- ½ cup of spreadable unsalted butter
- 1 medium egg
- 1 cup of brown sugar
- 1 ⅔ cups of all-purpose flour, sifted
- ¼ cup of milk
- 1 teaspoon vanilla
- 1 teaspoon of baking powder
- 15 large gumdrops, chopped finely

DIRECTIONS:

1. Preheat the oven at 400F/195C.
2. Combine the sugar, butter and egg until creamy.
3. Add the milk and vanilla and stir well.
4. Combine the flour with the baking powder in a different bowl. Incorporate to the sugar, butter mixture, and stir.
5. Add the gumdrops and place the mixture in the fridge for half an hour.
6. Drop the dough with tablespoonful into a lightly greased baking or cookie sheet.
7. Bake for 10-12 minutes or until golden brown in color.

Nutrition: *Calories: 102.17 kcal Carbohydrate: 16.5 g Protein: 0.86 g Sodium: 23.42 mg Potassium: 45 mg Phosphorus: 32.15 mg Dietary Fiber: 0.13 g Fat: 4 g*

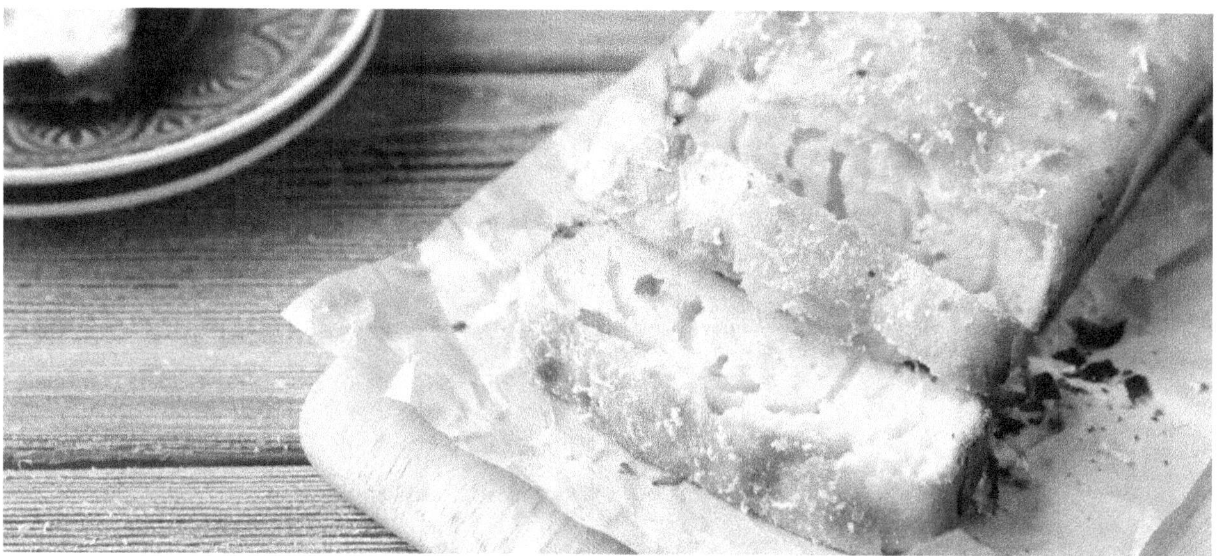

POUND CAKE WITH PINEAPPLE

INGREDIENTS:

- 3 cups of all-purpose flour, sifted
- 3 cups of sugar
- 1 ½ cups of butter
- 6 whole eggs and 3 egg whites
- 1 teaspoon of vanilla extract
- 1 10. ounce can of pineapple chunks, rinsed and crushed (keep juice aside).
- For glaze:
- 1 cup of sugar
- 1 stick of unsalted butter or margarine
- Reserved juice from the pineapple

DIRECTIONS:

1. Preheat the oven at 350F/180C.
2. Beat the sugar and the butter with a hand mixer until creamy and smooth.
3. Slowly add the eggs (one or two every time) and stir well after pouring each egg.
4. Add the vanilla extract, follow up with the flour and stir well.
5. Add the drained and chopped pineapple.
6. Pour the mixture into a greased cake tin and bake for 45-50 minutes.
7. In a small saucepan, combine the sugar with the butter and pineapple juice. Stir every few seconds and bring to boil. Cook until you get a creamy to thick glaze consistency.
8. Pour the glaze over the cake while still hot.
9. Let cook for at least 10 seconds and serve.

Nutrition: *Calories: 407.4 kcal Carbohydrate: 79 g Protein: 4.25 g Sodium: 118.97 mg Potassium: 180.32 mg Phosphorus: 66.37 mg Dietary Fiber: 2.25 g Fat: 16.48 g*

APPLE

CRUNCH PIE

INGREDIENTS:

- 4 large tart apples, peeled, seeded and sliced
- ½ cup of white all-purpose flour
- ⅓ cup margarine
- 1 cup of sugar
- ¾ cup of rolled oat flakes

- ½ teaspoon of ground nutmeg

DIRECTIONS:

1. Preheat the oven to 375F/180C.
2. Place the apples over a lightly greased square pan (around 7 inches).
3. Mix the rest of the ingredients in a medium bowl with and spread the batter over the apples.
4. Bake for 30-35 minutes or until the top crust has gotten golden brown.
5. Serve hot.

Nutrition: *Calories: 261.9 kcal Carbohydrate: 47.2 g Protein: 1.5 g Sodium: 81 mg Potassium: 123.74 mg Phosphorus: 35.27 mg Dietary Fiber: 2.81 g Fat: 7.99 g*

CHOCOLATE GELATIN MOUSSE

INGREDIENTS:

- 1 teaspoon stevia
- 1/2 teaspoon gelatin
- 1/4 cup milk
- 1/2 cup chocolate chips
- 1 teaspoon vanilla
- 1/2 cup heavy cream, whipped

DIRECTIONS:

1. Whisk the stevia with the gelatin and milk in a saucepan and cook up to a boil.
2. Stir in the chocolate and vanilla then mix well until it has completely melted.
3. Beat the cream in a mixer until fluffy then fold in the chocolate mixture.
4. Mix it gently with a spatula then transfer to the serving bowl.
5. Refrigerate the dessert for 4 hours.
6. Serve.

Nutrition: *Calories 200 Total Fat 12.1g Saturated Fat 8g Cholesterol 27mg Sodium 31mg Carbohydrate 4.7g Dietary Fiber 0.7g Sugars 0.8g Protein 3.2g Calcium 68mg Phosphorous 120mg Potassium 100mg*

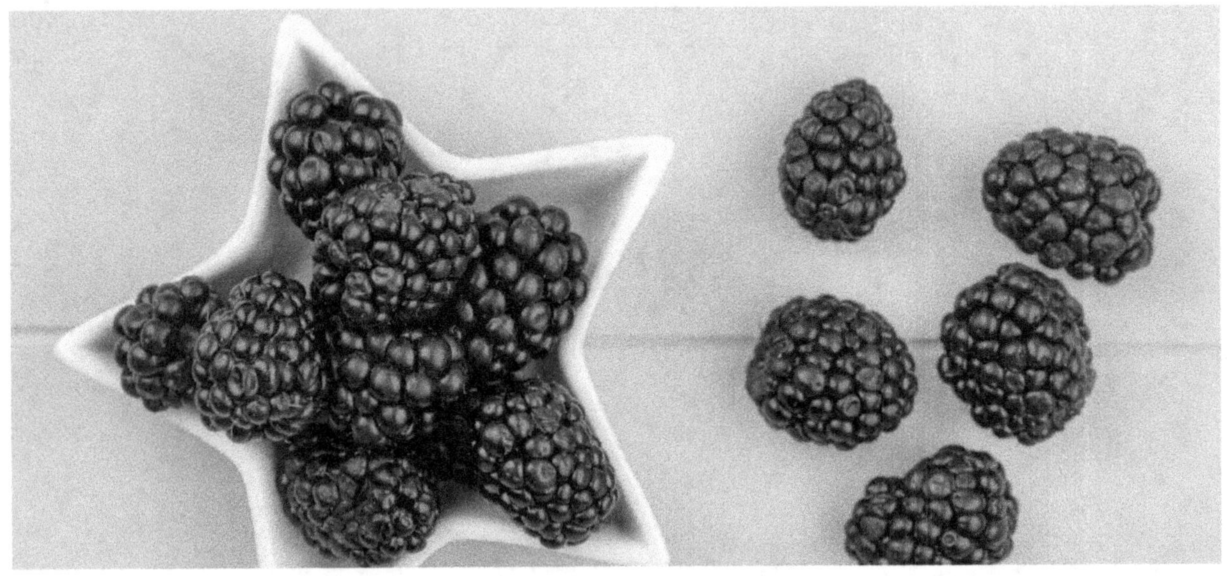

BLACKBERRY CREAM CHEESE PIE

INGREDIENTS:

- 1/3 cup butter, unsalted
- 4 cups blackberries
- 1 teaspoon stevia
- 1 cup flour
- 1/2 teaspoon baking powder
- 3/4 cup cream cheese

DIRECTIONS:

1. Switch your gas oven to 375 degrees F to preheat.
2. Layer a 2-quart baking dish with melted butter.
3. Mix the blackberries with stevia in a small bowl.
4. Beat the remaining ingredients in a mixer until they form a smooth batter.
5. Evenly spread this pie batter in the prepared baking dish and top it with blackberries.
6. Bake the blackberry pie for about 45 minutes in the preheated oven.
7. Slice and serve once chilled.

Nutrition: *Calories 239 Total Fat 8.4g Saturated Fat 4.9g Cholesterol 20mg Sodium 63mg Carbohydrate 26.2g Dietary Fiber 4.5g Sugars 15.1g Protein 2.8g Calcium 67mg Phosphorous 105mg Potassium 170mg*

APPLE CINNAMON PIE

INGREDIENTS:

- Apple Filling:
- 9 cups apples, peeled, cored and sliced
- 1 tablespoon stevia
- 1/3 cup all-purpose flour
- 2 tablespoons lemon juice
- 1 teaspoon ground cinnamon
- 2 tablespoons butter
- Pie Dough:
- 2 1/4 cups all-purpose flour
- 1 teaspoon stevia
- 1 1/2 sticks unsalted butter
- 6 oz. cream cheese
- 3 tablespoons cold heavy whipping cream
- Water, if needed

DIRECTIONS:

1. Start by preheating your gas oven at 425 degrees F.
2. Mix the apple slices with cinnamon, 1 tablespoon of butter, lemon juice, flour and stevia in a bowl and keep it aside covered.
3. Whisk the flour with stevia, butter, cream cheese and cream in mixing bowl to form the dough.
4. If the dough is too dry, slowly add some water to make a smooth dough ball.
5. Cut the dough into two equal-size pieces and spread them into a 9-inch sheet.
6. Place one of the sheets at the bottom of a 9-inch pie pan.
7. Evenly spread the apples in this pie shell and add a tablespoon of butter over it.
8. Cover the apple filling with the second sheet of the dough and pinch down the edges.
9. Make 1-inch deep cuts on top of the pie and bake for about 50 minutes until golden.
10. Slice and serve.

Nutrition: *Calories 303 Total Fat 8.8g Saturated Fat 5.3g Cholesterol 26mg Sodium 30mg Carbohydrate 21.7g Dietary Fiber 4.8g Sugars 19.6g Protein 4.2g Calcium 21mg Phosphorous 381mg Potassium 229mg*

MAPLE CRISP BARS

INGREDIENTS:

- 1/3 cup butter
- 1 cup brown Swerve
- 1 teaspoon maple extract
- 1/2 cup maple syrup
- 8 cups puffed rice cereal

DIRECTIONS:

1. Mix the butter with Swerve, maple extract, and syrup in a saucepan over moderate heat.
2. Cook by slowly stirring this mixture for 5 minutes then toss in the rice cereal.
3. Mix well, then press this cereal mixture in a 13x9 inches baking dish.
4. Refrigerate the mixture for 2 hours then cut into 20 bars. Serve

Nutrition: *Calories 107 Total Fat 3.1g Saturated Fat 0.5g Cholesterol 0mg Sodium 36mg Carbohydrate 10.6g Dietary Fiber 0.1g Sugars 5.4g Protein 0.4g Calcium 7mg Phosphorous 233mg Potassium 24mg*

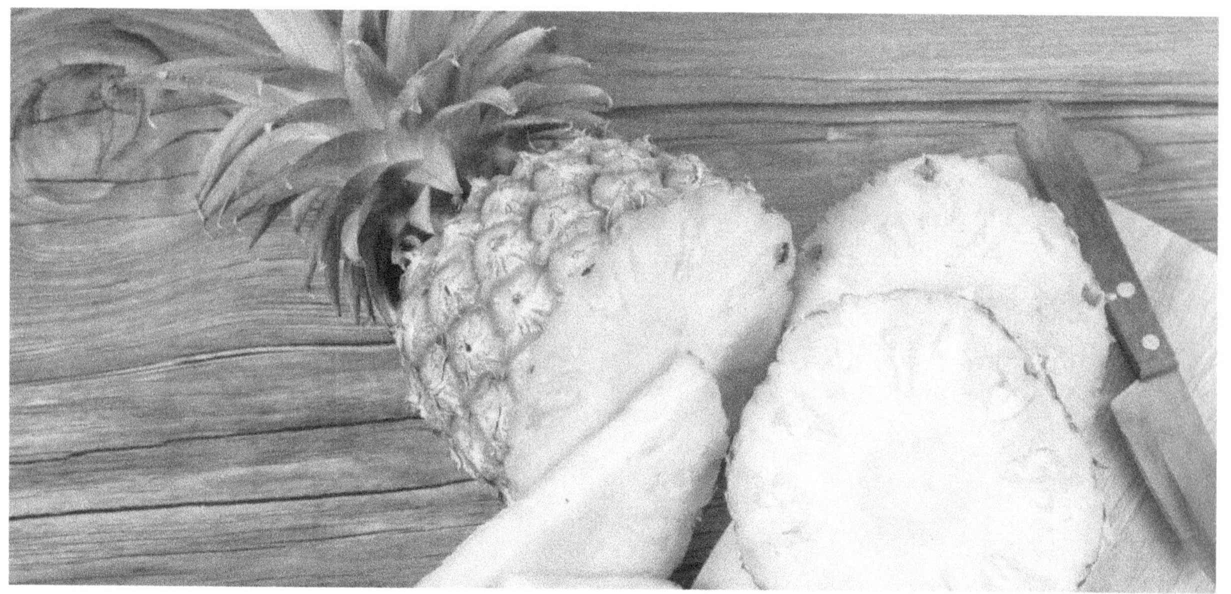

PINEAPPLE GELATIN PIE

INGREDIENTS:

- 2/3 cup graham cracker crumbs
- 2 1/2 tablespoons butter, melted
- 1 (20-oz) can crushed pineapple, juice packed
- 1 small gelatin pack
- 1 tablespoon lemon juice
- 2 egg whites, pasteurized
- 1/4 teaspoon cream of tartar

DIRECTIONS:

1. Whisk the crumbs with the butter in a bowl then spread them onto an 8-inch pie plate.
2. Bake the crust for 5 minutes at 425 degrees F.
3. Meanwhile, mix the pineapple juice with the gelatin in a saucepan.
4. Place it over low heat then add the pineapple and lemon juice. Mix well.
5. Beat the cream of tartar and egg whites in a mixer until creamy.
6. Add the cooked pineapple mixture then mix well.
7. Spread this filling in the baked crust.
8. Refrigerate the pie for 4 hours then slice.
9. Serve.

Nutrition: *Calories 106 Total Fat 4.2g Saturated Fat 0.6g Cholesterol 0mg Sodium 117mg Carbohydrate 14.5g Dietary Fiber 0.5g Sugars 9.4g Protein 2.2g Calcium 3mg Phosphorous 231mg Potassium 33mg*

CHERRY PIE DESSERT

INGREDIENTS:

- 1/2 cup butter, unsalted
- 2 eggs
- 1 cup granulated Swerve
- 1 cup sour cream
- 1 teaspoon vanilla
- 2 cups all-purpose flour
- 1 teaspoon baking powder
- 1 teaspoon baking soda
- 20 oz. cherry pie filling

DIRECTIONS:

1. First, begin by setting your gas oven at 350 degrees F.
2. Soften the butter first, then beat it with the cream eggs, Swerve, vanilla, and sour cream in a mixer.
3. Separately mix the flour with the baking soda and baking powder.
4. Add this mixture to the egg mixture and mix well until smooth.
5. Spread the batter evenly in a 9x13 inch baking pan.
6. Bake the pie for 40 minutes in the oven until golden from the surface.
7. Slice and serve with cherry pie filling on top.

Nutrition: *Calories 470 Total Fat 19g Saturated Fat 11.4g Cholesterol 84mg Sodium 285mg Carbohydrate 43.2g Dietary Fiber 1.3g Sugars 14.9g Protein 5.9g Calcium 82mg Phosphorous 249mg Potassium 232mg*

STRAWBERRY PIZZA

INGREDIENTS:

- Crust:
- 1 cup flour
- 1/4 cup Swerve
- 1/2 cup butter
- Filling:
- 8 oz. cream cheese, softened
- 1/2 teaspoon vanilla
- ¾ tablespoon stevia
- 2 cups sliced strawberries

DIRECTIONS:

1. Mix the flour with the Swerve, butter, and enough water to make a dough.
2. Spread this dough evenly in a pie pan.
3. Bake the crust for 15 minutes at 350 degrees F.
4. Beat the cream cheese with the stevia and vanilla in a mixer until fluffy.
5. Spread this cream cheese filling in the crust and top it with strawberries.

6. Serve.

Nutrition: *Calories 235 Total Fat 14.5g Saturated Fat 9g Cholesterol 41mg Sodium 112mg Carbohydrate 12.8g Dietary Fiber 1g Sugars 9.3g Protein 2.8g Calcium 25mg Phosphorous 236mg Potassium 84mg*

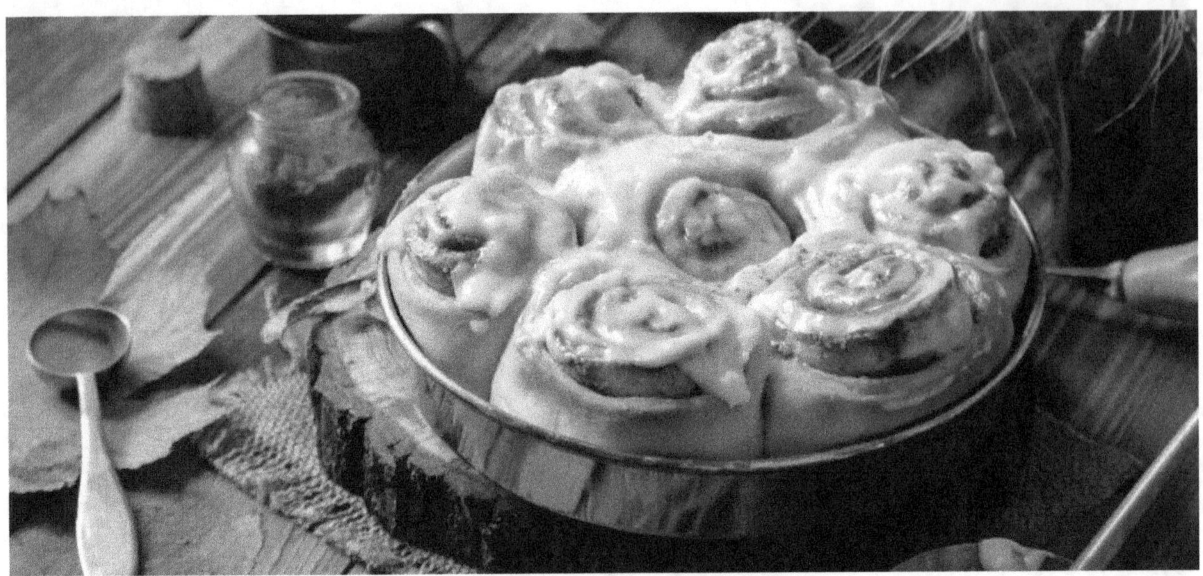

PUMPKIN CINNAMON ROLL

INGREDIENTS:

- Dough:
- 1 1/2 cups milk
- 1/2 cup olive oil
- 1/2 cup granulated Swerve
- 2 1/4 teaspoons active dry yeast
- 1 cup pumpkin puree
- 4 1/2 cups flour
- 1/2 teaspoon ground cinnamon
- 1/4 teaspoon ground ginger
- 1/4 teaspoon ground nutmeg
- 1/2 teaspoon baking powder
- 1/2 teaspoon baking soda
- Melted butter, for buttering pans
- Filling:
- 1/2 cup butter, melted
- 1/2 cup brown Swerve
- 1/2 cup granulated Swerve
- 1/2 teaspoon cinnamon
- 1/2 teaspoon ground ginger
- 1/4 teaspoon ground nutmeg

DIRECTIONS:

1. Switch on your gas oven and let it preheat at 375 degrees F.
2. Whisk all the ingredients for the dough in a mixing bowl.
3. Spread the dough in a loaf pan into a ½-inch layer and bake it for 15 minutes.
4. Meanwhile, whisk all the ingredients for the filling in a bowl.
5. Place the baked cake in a serving plate and top it with the prepared filling.
6. Roll the cake and slice it.
7. Serve.

Nutrition: *Calories 201 Total Fat 9.2g Saturated Fat 3.7g Cholesterol 12mg Sodium 63mg Carbohydrate 14.9g Dietary Fiber 1g Sugars 3.1g Protein 3.2g Calcium 32mg Phosphorous 277mg Potassium 91mg*

Conclusion

Kidney disease now ranks as the 18th deadliest condition in the world. In the United States alone, it is reported that over 600,000 Americans succumb to kidney failure.

These stats are alarming, which is why, it is necessary to take proper care of your kidneys, starting with a kidney-friendly diet.

In this Book, you will learn how to create dishes that are healthy, delicious and easy on your kidneys.

These recipes are ideal whether you have been diagnosed with a kidney problem or you want to prevent any kidney issue.

With regards to your wellbeing and health, it's a smart thought to see your doctor as frequently as conceivable to ensure you don't run into preventable issues that you needn't get. The kidneys are your body's toxin channel (just like the liver), cleaning the blood of remote substances and toxins that are discharged from things like preservatives in food & other toxins.

At the point when you eat flippantly and fill your body with toxins, either from nourishment, drinks (liquor or alcohol for instance) or even from the air you inhale (free radicals are in the sun and move through your skin, through messy air, and numerous food sources contain them). Your body additionally will in general convert numerous things that appear to be benign until your body's organs convert them into things like formaldehyde because of a synthetic response and transforming phase.

One case of this is a large portion of those diet sugars utilized in diet soft drinks for instance, Aspartame transforms into Formaldehyde in the body. These toxins must be expelled or they can prompt ailment, renal (kidney) failure, malignant growth, & various other painful problems.

This isn't a condition that occurs without any forethought it is a dynamic issue and in that it very well may be both found early and treated, diet changed, and settling what is causing the issue is conceivable. It's conceivable to have partial renal failure yet, as a rule; it requires some time (or downright awful diet for a short time) to arrive at absolute renal failure. You would prefer not to reach total renal failure since this will require standard dialysis treatments to save your life.

Dialysis treatments explicitly clean the blood of waste and toxins in the blood utilizing a machine in light of the fact that your body can no longer carry out the responsibility. Without treatments, you could die a very painful death. Renal failure can be the consequence of long haul diabetes, hypertension, unreliable diet, and can stem from other health concerns.

A renal diet is tied in with directing the intake of protein and phosphorus in your eating routine. Restricting your sodium intake is likewise significant. By controlling these two variables you can control the vast majority of the toxins/waste made by your body and thus this enables your kidney to 100% function. In the event that you get this early enough and truly moderate your diets with extraordinary consideration, you could avert all-out renal failure. In the event that you get this early, you can take out the issue completely.